THE MONKEYS in MY DREAMS

HEALING GENERATIONAL TRAUMA THROUGH LOVE, HOPE & FORGIVENESS

Pauline,
Wishing you love, hope & forgiveness!
Hopefully this brings back good memories!
[illegible]

The Monkeys in My Dreams - Healing Generational Trauma Through Love, Hope & Forgiveness

Written by Anne-Marie Bacon

A Division of Anita Sechesky – Living Without Limitations Inc.

LWL PUBLISHING HOUSE uses American Standard English in all of its publications.

The diary entries at the beginning of the chapters have been left unaltered to retain the authenticity of the author's voice.

LWL PUBLISHING HOUSE
Email: lwlclienthelp@gmail.com
Website: www.lwlpublishinghouse.com

The Monkeys in My Dreams - Healing Generational Trauma Through Love, Hope & Forgiveness

Anita Sechesky – Living Without Limitations Inc.
ISBN 978-1-988867-35-9

Book Cover Design: N. Sechesky
Inside Layout: LWL PUBLISHING HOUSE Editorial Team

LWL
PUBLISHING HOUSE

Table of Contents

Part One

HISTORY REPEATS ITSELF

Part Two

LOVE, MARRIAGE, BETRAYALS, ADVENTURE

Part Three

TRAGEDY, SADNESS, JOY, PEACE, ENDINGS

Legal Disclaimer

The Monkeys in My Dreams - Healing Generational Trauma Through Love, Hope & Forgiveness does not substitute any form of professional counsel such as a Psychologist, Physician, Life Coach, or Counselor. The contents and information provided does not constitute professional or legal advice in any way, shape, or form.

All chapters are written at the discretion of and with the full accountability of the author. Anita Sechesky – Living Without Limitations Inc. or LWL PUBLISHING HOUSE is not liable or responsible for any of the specific details, descriptions of people, places or things, personal interpretations, stories and experiences contained within. The Publisher is not liable for any misrepresentations, false or unknown statements, actions, or judgments made by the author of this book, who is responsible for her own material and has shared her information in good faith to encourage others.

Any decisions you make and the outcomes thereof are entirely your own doing. Under no circumstances can you hold the author, LWL PUBLISHING HOUSE, or Anita Sechesky – Living Without Limitations Inc. liable for any actions that you take.

You agree not to hold the author, LWL PUBLISHING HOUSE, or Anita Sechesky – Living Without Limitations Inc. liable for any loss or expense incurred by you, as a result of materials, advice, coaching or mentoring offered within.

The information offered in this book is intended to be general information with respect to general life issues. Information is offered in good faith; however, you are under no obligation to use this information.

Nothing contained in this book shall be considered legal, financial,

Dedication

For Mom; may your stories inspire forgiveness and healing. To Denis and our daughters; if it weren't for you and your everlasting support, I may never have finished it. To my grandchildren; may you discover your family history.

Foreword

Lasting relationships create the essence of what makes us who we are. The closer the connection, the stronger the emotions involved and the degree of impact it makes in the lives of those we choose to form those very special relationships with. Therefore, the dynamics of family ties make these relationships even more significant in how they impact the generations to come.

Have you ever witnessed the breakdown of any relationship? It can start from misunderstandings, jealousy, misguided information, abuse, false witness, lack of sensitivity, preconceived ideas, biases, false representations, grudges, lack of insight, unforgiveness, loss of trust or respect, pride, judgmental or critical perceptions, or an unwillingness to give another person a fair consideration to prove themselves right and honorable.

As an individual who has worked with hundreds of people in the health care industry as well as interacting on a regular basis with coaching clients and new authors, I can honestly say a communication breakdown often happens when there is a heightened expectation from one party that is not usually brought about until a lack of "some kind of perception" is revealed or exposed. This is not always the case unless there is deep thought into the matter at hand. In most cases, the shifts in a relationship often lead to a gap of misunderstandings and unresolved emotions which is the usual downside of more personal relationships such as family, and siblings in particular. Many people do not seek outside support or counseling when important issues come up and as a result, years of missed opportunities go by. It's either a death, a wedding, or a birth that finally bring favorable circumstances for healing and forgiveness. But if the pain or emotional damage is deep, there is usually no resolve in the matter. I trust that you will find some inspiration and insight within these pages to help you with your personal situation or communication breakdowns, and you won't let your relationships get lost for too long.

It has been a pleasure to work with Anne-Marie and to help her articulate the language of healing love with the respect and thoughtfulness a story like hers needed. I'm also grateful we captured what was requested by her late mother about some of their significant and traumatic life experiences for their future generations, to help bring about healing and unity in the years to come. You will find that in reading this insightful book about Anne-Marie's family dynamics, spanning several generations, that you just can't avoid the interactions that come into play within close relations. Because of her commitment and dedication to getting this book published in less than a year, we are proud that Anne-Marie kept her promise to her mother.

Remember that regardless of what anyone else's opinions or feelings may be, your state of healthy peace, forgiveness, and happiness should be of utmost consideration as you choose to put others in a place of peaceful resolve. As you read and learn about the author's life and the experiences she and her loved ones faced, we hope that you will also find the courage and discover your voice to release the healing you need to live the life of adventure and vitality you deserve with those closest to you.

In Peace & Gratitude,

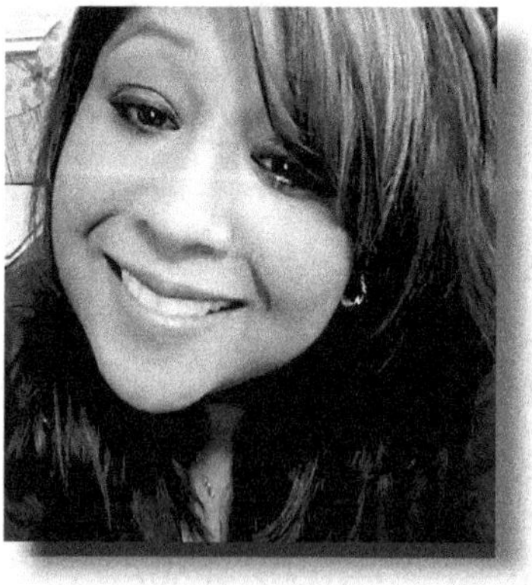

Anita Sechesky

RN, Holistic Book Writing Coach, Founder, Owner, CEO & Publisher at LWL PUBLISHING HOUSE

Email: lwlclienthelp@gmail.com

Website: www.lwlpublishinghouse.com

Website: www.anitasechesky.com

LWL PUBLISHING HOUSE (Facebook Business page)
www.facebook.com/lwlpublishinghouse

LIVING WITHOUT LIMITATIONS in PRINT (Facebook Business page)
www.facebook.com/AnitaSechesky

Anita's Private Facebook group: LIVING WITHOUT LIMITATIONS in PRINT www.facebook.com/groups/LivingWithoutLimitationsInPrint

LinkedIn: https://ca.linkedin.com/in/asechesky

Twitter: https://twitter.com/nursie4u

Acknowledgments

To start with, if it weren't for my mother this book would never have happened. Her stories are what inspired me to begin. My promise to her, to finish it, is what kept me going.

Next, I have to thank Andrew McLeod for keeping a straight face after reading my very first draft of the manuscript. He gave me some difficult advice and I am forever grateful. Following in his footsteps, France Foster helped me find my way to LWL PUBLISHING HOUSE. Thanks to both of you.

At LWL PUBLISHING HOUSE, I was welcomed with open arms by the Publisher, Anita Sechesky. She facilitated my learning curve in writing about the sensitive topics within my book, helped me develop the outline, and has been amazing with her support of my vision for this publication. I owe a huge debt of gratitude to Anita and her team at LWL PUBLISHING HOUSE for all of the final editing, formatting, and graphic designs. Thank you so much, Anita.

I would be remiss if I didn't thank all my friends and co-workers who have helped me process ideas for this or that. Bouncing thoughts off all of you has been very helpful and I thank you. I especially need to thank Anita and Paulette, my Ya-Ya's who have been hearing about this book for a very long time. Finally you get to read it! Thank you for never giving up on me. Merci.

To my aunts, uncles, and cousins who all told pretty amazing stories that helped me fill in some blanks. Thank you to everyone.

To my siblings who have shared or clarified intimate stories with me cause you're all mostly older than me and remember them more clearly. Thank you all for your help. To my sisters Colette and Monique,

I need to especially thank you for your endless support, patience, and love. Without you two, I'd have given up long ago. Heartfelt thanks to you both.

To my daughters, my love and appreciation for you both are bottomless. Your encouragement, candid honesty, and integrity kept me on the straight and narrow. Much love and thanks to the two of you and your amazing families.

To my dearest Denis, my sweetie. Your allegiance to me and your belief in this book has not gone unnoticed. You have to be the most unflappable man alive! I have been talking about this book for eons and through it all, you championed it and me. To see it to completion with you by my side is surreal. Thank you, thank you, thank you, Denis.

Introduction

The Monkeys in My Dreams is a book that crosses generations, proving that in spite of trauma, we can overcome; we can be kind and loving; we can be successful!

There are stories that may alarm you, entertain you, or make you laugh or cry! There are accounts of love, tragedy, infidelity, generosity, and most importantly forgiveness.

I have known since I was a child that I'd write this book and that the title would be *The Monkeys in My Dreams*. I didn't know how or when I'd start but I knew I'd write it. Then, with what began as an important conversation with my mother, I learned so much more about my family history. I started taking careful notes, recording in journals, and eventually started writing.

A few years later I would move a couple of hundred kilometers away from home and Mom, after which we began our Sunday morning ritual of phone calls. It was our special time: Mom with her coffee and me with my tea. We'd cover all the minutiae of our week and then I'd get my history lesson. At times I was appalled – this was my family history, our legacy! I hope you'll find these stories as interesting as I have.

My mother trusted me with her innermost feelings and was very open about her family history. Her pain was as raw as a gaping wound. She wanted to share this very personal story as she thought that maybe someday it might save another child from the same fate she suffered. She was determined that her children, and her family, would never suffer abuse at her hands or on her watch.

I wanted her to share her story so that she could unburden herself and in doing so, she was miraculously able to forgive her abusers. She had every reason to be bitter, angry, and mean but she chose to be kind, loving, generous and made forgiveness her life's mission.

My mother was adamant that I publish this book. On her deathbed, she maintained the importance of this. She wanted people to learn from her history and wanted to give her pain meaning. There had to be a reason she went through all she did!

Over the years I've connected with so many people whose experiences resonated with mine. I find it interesting that these families all have dynamics of their own but similar pain is shared by them all. My hope is that in reading my book, it will help you process your own emotional healing by seeing the parallels of our stories.

It rarely is pretty when delving into the past. It can be painful for some and bring up anguished feelings for others. Mom felt it was our responsibility to use these dreadful experiences to bring about change. If we sweep all this under a rug, it's going to get lumpy and eventually someone is going to trip on that rug!

I want to be clear that this is not a revenge book. There is no malice intended. My mother and father were born in wartime. Society was different, people were suffering, life was hard, and we didn't have TV talk show hosts to tell us what was right or wrong!

I want this book to empower people, to help them sort out their feelings, to give them the strength to move on from any strained relationships in their lives regardless if those people are still part of their lives or not.

You will read about my father. I want you to know that in spite of his faults, I loved him. In order for me to forgive him, I had to come to a place where I realized that my father did the best he could with what he knew. He had no idea how his actions affected his family. By forgiving him, it has allowed me to unload the burden that I carried around for so many years.

When my mother was on her deathbed, I asked her what she wanted most for her family. Her reply was that she wanted us to forgive one another. Mom was very proud of her family; it was always so meaningful to her that her family not be divided. I am happy to report that we are working on this and I know Mom is up there nudging us all on. She is smiling.

With this book, I not only want to be a historian, but I also want to be the change-maker in you! I want you to read my book and take your life back! No more grudges hauling around; no more baggage! Forgive those that hurt you – you'll see how it frees you! Since I chose to forgive those who hurt me, things started shifting in my life. I am happier, more focused, and able to write again. I no longer let it consume me.

I want you, the readers, to be brave, bold, and go out and conquer the world! Stop talking about the hurt and betrayals and set it all free. You deserve peace. Forgive those that need forgiving. Mom would be so proud of you as well!

Anne-Marie

Part One

HISTORY REPEATS ITSELF

Chapter One

YOUNG LOVE - 1980

September 15, 1978

Dear Diary,

Do you believe in the stars sending you love? Cowabanga Dude! I met the cutest guy tonight! His intense blue eyes had me at Hello! I need to get to know him better, no...way better, what's a better word for better? I think I'll ask him to my brother's wedding as my chaperone. Here's hoping Dear Diary.

July 22, 1979

Dear Diary,

My sweetie Denis and I are just motoring along! He's the best thing that has ever happened to me. He's a great listener which is good because you know I'm a bit of a talker! He's bloody adorable, but has this tough guy kinda look but he doesn't have me fooled one bit. I feel so safe with him. We just can't seem to get enough of each other, I love this guy so much! I really need to get to the doctors and talk about birth control soon Diary.

February 7, 1980

Dear Diary,

Good news/bad news. Good news, I got accepted today to the college in Toronto for the foodservice program. Bad news, I will not be able to accept. This makes me incredibly sad as everything changed the minute I found out I was pregnant. On that note, I finally had the guts to talk to Mom, and I told her the news today. I was mostly concerned that she'd kick me out of the house as they haven't exactly been the most supportive parents of late. My sister is living at a YMCA in Windsor (while my parents live in a five-bedroom lake house) because she can't afford an apartment. She is one tough sister! As it turns out my parents are being supportive of me. Mom said she will help me however I need. My mother, though, was more concerned about Dad's reaction than anything. He has some nerve judging me considering what he's been up to! Like Dad is the poster boy of purity, give me a break! I know where he's at every night. He might fool Mom and perhaps my siblings, but not me. Does he not know what I know about him and my aunt? Until next time, Diary.

The gymnasium was dark, there were disco balls creating cool shadows on the gym walls, and Rod Stewart's *"Da Ya Think I'm Sexy?"* was blaring from the speakers. I looked around for my friends and they had vanished! They had all found someone to either dance with or were snuggling up to someone! Hooray, I thought, now what do I do? I went out into the hall, headed for the canteen/snack bar, and unknowingly kicked a pop can that was lying on the ground. This bored-looking guy across the hall, dressed in tight-fitting Levis and an Oakland Raiders Jersey with #49 on it, kicked the can back. He had this "I dare you" look on his face, so I stopped in my tracks, looked into those incredible blue eyes, and kicked it right back with a tiny little grin!

You see...I have four brothers, and nobody intimidates me! Next thing you know, we are kicking this can back and forth and giggling about it until a teacher came around and picked it up while giving both of us a dirty look. I guess we were so wrapped up in this "can passing" that we were oblivious to the racket we were causing. I'm not sure if Denis and I spoke much to each other that night, but we did share a laugh about the pop can and we both moved on.

On the way home that night, I told my friends I knew who I'd ask to chaperone me to my brother's wedding. "His name is Denis. He's a football player," I said. They all shouted their "woo-hoos" and replied that I should definitely ask him out because he was so cute. This was very important when you're sixteen! I'm sure if Denis were to talk of our first meeting, he'd call me a firecracker or something of that sort.

The following week, I finally got up the nerve to ask him to chaperone me to my brother's wedding. He said he didn't know if he could or not and that I had put him on the spot. I replied with, "I need an answer, yes or no." And since I was feeling lucky, I pushed a bit more than I needed to. He said ***Yes!*** I was very happy and ran off to tell my friends. Even way back then, I knew how to close a deal.

My brother's wedding was our first official date and because I was standing in the wedding, Denis was accompanied by a couple of my friends and their dates. They had dinner at their own table as I fulfilled my junior bridesmaid duties. They were especially keen on the roasted chicken that was served, not to mention all the other delicious foods! Eventually, I was able to join them at their table and take in all the fun. Drinks, dancing, and whooping it up, we all had a great time!

After that night Denis and I began dating like our lives depended on it. We just could not get enough of each other. He was a great listener and I a great talker! He loved a lot of the same movies as I, I tolerated all the football watching, I went to his hockey games, he came to my baseball games, and time was flying. We were getting very serious, talking about the future, and planning a life together. It just seemed like we couldn't see a future without each other.

We discussed going to post-secondary school together in Toronto. I would go to a well-known college and Denis would attend a technology institute. I went to the doctor's to get on the pill as we didn't want to mess things up. Alas, my timing was off and I was too late. I was pregnant. "Dear Lord, how will I tell my mother. Oh boy, oh boy, this will go over like a lead balloon."

I went to bed that night and wrote in my journal for the first time in a long time. Sometimes I find writing helps me process things.

Tomorrow I will talk to Mom.

The wind howled outside the windows as I tried to quiet my mind. It was a very cold February day. Our home was a beautiful big two-story house on the shore of Lake St. Clair in a small sleepy village called Stoney Point in Ontario, Canada. The year was 1980 and I was sitting on the carpeted floor of our large TV room, leaning back against my mother's black leather reclining chair. My sizable family often gathered around the 26-inch television, which was considered a large model back then.

The house smelled of chicken and sliders, a comforting food if there ever was one. We were watching *The Mike Douglas Show*. My mother, having worked all day, was now folding laundry and taking in Mike's comments while giving her version of advice as well. Doubtless, she'd have advice for me too after what I had to say.

I kept thinking, "Just tell her!" Finally, feeling as if I was ripping off a three-day-old bandage, I said, "Mom, I have something to talk to you about."

"I know you do. You want to go on the pill," Mom declared with certainty, oblivious to my reality.

"I wish we'd had that talk a few months ago!" I sighed.

Mom understood immediately that I was pregnant. I told her I was due early August. Her first reaction surprised me.

"I'm not going to be the one telling your father!" she warned. "You'll have to do that dirty job on your own!"

I knew "it" was about to hit the fan in a big way. I'm the youngest girl of eight children and my father would not like a daughter of his being shamed like this. I finally braced myself to go and face him when Mom suddenly changed her mind. She went to deliver the news. I felt such relief and love for my mother at that moment. She was taking yet another bullet for one of her kids and I felt like such a coward!

My mother drove to the Stoney Point Tavern, a restaurant that my parents owned and operated. You'd find my father there every day of the week. He was likely in his office watching *The Mike Douglas Show* too and pretending to be working. Mom walked in and told him she had something to tell him.

"Can't it wait?" he asked. "This is an important program!"

"No, it can't," answered Mom. "This is more important." She told him I was pregnant.

"You're sure?" said Dad, after a momentous silence.

"Oooh, yes, we're sure," Mom confirmed. I've never really been told the whole story of his reaction, but my imagination and my experience of Dad's response to other previously bad news was a tip-off that he likely flung quite a few cuss words before finally saying, "Well? What is she going to do?"

Mom came back home after speaking with Dad, if I can really use the word "speaking" in a case such as this! She sat with me and said she'd call all seven of my siblings and spread the word. This was very gracious of Mom since she knew how hard it would be for me to do this.

My family's reaction was instantaneous. To this day, I'm still shocked at the unconditional support they offered. My brothers and sisters either came over or called me and talked on forever about how they'd help; they were all true to their word. Through all these years, they have never let me or my family down.

My mom's main concern was for my child not to suffer a terrible upbringing like hers. Essentially, Mom had never told me anything about her childhood, so I asked her to explain and she proceeded to tell me in great detail. She was brought up as a stepchild in her family and never knew her birth father or even his name. "That's not going to happen to your child!" she announced. I assured her that none of that would happen.

I then called Denis, my sweetie, to let him know how it all went. He had been anxious for my call and nervous about my family's reaction. He thought he'd be banned from the house for good. On the contrary, my siblings contacted him and told Denis to ask if he needed anything at all.

Denis and I talked endlessly about keeping the baby – there was never a question really. We considered how we would support our child. Denis had just turned eighteen and I was close behind him. I had just completed my high school diploma requirements and would graduate in June. I'd received my acceptance to the college in Toronto for their food and beverage program the previous Thursday which was, ironically, the same day I got confirmation from the doctor about my pregnancy. Could I go to school and be a young, first-time mother at the same time? Denis himself was intending to go on to post-secondary education and was working full-time at a bicycle shop to build up his funds to do just that. We had some big decisions to make and needed to find answers, and soon.

The incoming phone calls were unending, especially from so-called friends, some of whom I'd never been very close to. One particular "friend" phoned on behalf of a group of acquaintances eager to know if I was, in fact, preggers. She must have drawn the short straw. "Yes, it is true," I told her and proceeded to listen to all her questions, the same ones that we were being asked over and over by everyone who called. "What will you do?" "Where will you live?" "Will you get married?" "How will you support a baby?" "Will you still go to school?" The questions went on and on and I was getting weary of them all plus being hit with the reality of what was happening to me!

Denis and I spent hours going over these questions ourselves. I knew for sure that abortion and adoption were not options for us. I realized this child was going to be special and that God had a plan for me, although it would've made things a lot easier if I knew what that plan might be. My mother had agreed that the baby and I could live at home until we had figured these things out. I didn't want to get married while I was pregnant, and I didn't want to hear for the rest of my life, "I only married you because you were pregnant!" Not that Denis would do that, but I didn't want to give him that opportunity. I was adamant about no wedding until after the baby was born, and besides, Denis hadn't even asked me yet!

As far as support, I would work like every other parent in this world has done that was necessary to support their child. I had no doubts that Denis would be there to help as well. I was completely naïve as to how hard it would be, but perhaps that was a good thing. I had no idea that a case of formula would cost me a day's wages or that babysitting fees would drain my checking account faster than I had thought possible.

School was a difficult decision. As far as I could see, there was no way to pay for that. Therefore, my education was going to be put on hold. I had no idea back then that I could have gotten loans and grants from the government to help pay for school, and that even childcare would have been covered. Instead, I just put that dream aside and went about my day-to-day life with a brave face. Looking back now, I think the truth was that I was trying to punish myself for getting into "trouble." If I were to do this all over again, I would spend the time and money to get an education. It is so valuable and opens many doors for you.

I hoped Denis would go to school, and he did, eventually. I gladly worked to help support the three of us throughout the time that he attended the technology institute. I had no doubt Denis would do the same once he had graduated. There wasn't any way for me to know this for sure, except that I felt it was true. He was loyal and never swayed from his obligations for one moment. Not once did he threaten to leave, even when the pregnancy hormones had me acting like a raving lunatic!

Chapter Two

MOM TELLS MEME D.

Dear Diary,

Whoa, today Mom called Meme D! It turns out that she was in a similar predicament to me, an unwed mother in 1935! Can you imagine the backlash, wow! I thought 1980 was bad, at least I had my sweetie to support me. Times were far different then, her father didn't take too kindly to the idea, I learned so much about my Mom's family today! Still, I think there's more to this story. Knowing my Meme, she would've married her boyfriend if she loved him......and what of Meme B's reaction?

Today I learned that Meme D. was in the same predicament back in her time; this makes me hopeful. If Meme were able to pull this off in 1935, then I should be able to do the same in 1980! I know with certainty that it won't be easy. It's strange how history has repeated itself.

My maternal grandmother, whom I called Meme D., was a wonderful woman that always had a smile on her face despite how her day may have been going. She was a shorter woman with a few extra pounds around the middle, "to keep her grounded" she'd say. She always had a lovely scent about her, no doubt from a beauty product as she had cases of samples from her old selling days. She was a great cook and could stretch a pound of ground meat like nobody I ever knew. She also was a great baker and made these peanut butter chews that'd put a smile on your face in spite of a bad day at school or work!

One of the first people my mother phoned regarding my pregnancy was Meme D. and her reaction was one of reverence. She told Mom how she herself had broken very similar news to her father, my great-grandfather exactly forty-five years before.

It was a cold, windy night during that February of 1935. Pepe B was still up and in the kitchen making himself a cuppa tea. Meme's sister was sitting in the stairwell waiting to talk to her father, Da or Pepe B. to me. She was very leery of this as she knew he wasn't going to be happy. She was about to announce her upcoming nuptials and her pregnancy. She sat on the stairs and waited for everyone to go to bed. Her sister, Meme D., was still up and she wondered what Meme D. was talking to Da about in the kitchen. Didn't Meme D. know she had news to share with him as well?

Da did not look happy, and when he stood up and shouted, "Who's the father of this child?!" Meme's sister instantly knew she was not about to make her own announcement that night. Meme D. ran past her sister in the stairwell and up to her room since she had refused to tell her father the identity of the baby's father.

All Meme knew was that she wanted to raise this child and be a good mother. She had heard of ways to get rid of a pregnancy but those went against her beliefs and morals, so that wasn't happening. When listening to this story, I couldn't help but feel ambivalence as here I was in the very same predicament...well almost. I knew the father and was glad to share that info. I could very well imagine how Meme D. was feeling since I was experiencing the same thing right then.

All of my life, I've remembered Meme D's father, Pepe B. as a fun kind of guy at all the New Year's parties. He and Meme B. would host this huge party with all their family. There would be close to 100 in attendance. We children would play in the stairwell as the basement was filled with the adults enjoying euchre, and smoking. Man oh man, there was a lot of smoking and drinking going on! This was usually the only time we would come as a family to visit them. I wasn't really fond of the bagpipers though as I thought of them as loud and a bit scary (today, I appreciate them, however). What I did like about the parties were the candy dishes! Meme had them set up all over the house. We would fill our pockets and head for the stairs to chat and catch up with our cousins while chomping on candy.

So hearing that Pepe B. was being strict came as a bit of a shock to me. If Pepe were alive today, I wonder if his reaction would have been different about this same situation. Would he be more supportive?

Meme's sister decided not to tell Da that night considering his reaction to Meme's news. Meme's sister had to learn that Meme D. was pregnant by hearing her tell their father. Why hadn't she confided in her? Then again, she hadn't yet shared her news with Meme D. either. They had lots of catching up to do.

Meme's sister went on to elope and get married. Meme D. and her boyfriend stood in for them as witnesses. Throughout the pregnancy Meme's boyfriend would come by to visit her but Pepe B. would not let him in. He was shunned from Meme D.'s life because the pregnancy was a disgrace to the family and in Pepe's eyes, it was this boyfriend's fault. Meme D. says she wanted to marry him but her father wouldn't allow it. It makes you wonder why she didn't do it regardless. Considering her sister was also pregnant, ran off, and got married, why didn't Meme? I think if she really loved him, she would have. That's my unprofessional opinion.

Meme's boyfriend went on working in Detroit but living in Windsor. He never married or had children but often inquired about Meme D. and her child – my mother.

Meme D. gave birth to a healthy little girl on September 27, 1935, and named her Beverley Mercedes. That beautiful baby would thirty years later become my mom!

After only a few weeks of recuperation, Meme D. ended up going back to work in Detroit where she was a housekeeper for a wealthy family. She would stay there all week while her mother and siblings cared for baby Bev.

So far, it was a good life for baby Bev: she was loved by her aunts and uncles, well-fed, and completely cared for while her mommy was working in Detroit. This beautiful baby was welcomed by a large devoted family and was loved deeply by them. Meme B, my great-grandmother was a colossal help to my grandmother, Meme D. She helped her daughter out as much as she could, while still not disobeying her husband, at least in public. I'm pretty sure I know where Mom's sass came from. Oh, how her family loved her sass.

But life would soon change for little Bev. Her new family wouldn't appreciate her sass near as much. She had a new reality coming soon: promises of a new daddy, don't quite meet the expectations of her dreams; sadly she will be so very disappointed.

Chapter Three

LIFE OF THE STEP-CHILD

Marriage Of Convenience

August 3, 1938

Dear Diary,

Today I could see Mom's pain when she shared the story of how Meme D. and Pepe D. met. Bloody Hell! So, because he needs a nanny, but was too cheap to get one, he gets a wife? Who does that? The only way for me to justify this is to think that times were different back then I suppose. Why did Meme D. think so little of herself that she would marry a man just because he needed a wife? From what I understand, they did not marry out of love; it was an arranged marriage that was all in his favour. If she wanted to give Mom a father, why not marry her boyfriend? I know Pepe D. wanted to gain a wife because a nanny can quit her job at any time, but it wasn't so easy for a wife to leave a man back then! I wonder, dear diary, did Meme have any clues when Pepe courted her, as to his personality? So by Mom marrying Pepe D., this makes Mom the unwanted step-child. No wonder she was disappointed when she found out I was pregnant. She was so worried my child would have a life like her own. I promised her that my daughter would not, and she won't. I cannot imagine the atrocities she lived through, it makes me so sad to hear these stories, yet I know it unburdens

Mom to talk about it. It certainly explains why she would not let us stay on overnight sleepovers with our cousins. If I could get in a time machine right here, right now, I'd have Mom explain to Dad on their honeymoon or even while dating, that she was abused as a little girl and that he'd need to be patient. If only we had a way of going back and setting things right, what a world we'd inhabit!

One afternoon, my Meme D. and a few of her friends were in the local pub owned by a family in Belle River. She was with one of her sisters who was dating the son of the family who owned the pub. While sitting together, her sister's boyfriend said to Meme D. that he knew of a man who needed a wife. Would she like to meet him? Her answer was yes, and the meeting was set up.

Pepe D. told her he was a widower. His wife had died during childbirth three years earlier. He was fifteen years older than Meme D. and had five children ranging in ages three to ten. Pepe D. was told by Children's Services that his current arrangement of having his son look after the smaller children while he worked was not appropriate, as his son was only ten years old and needed to be in school. Children's Services were going to remove the children if Pepe D. did not find either a nanny or a wife! The way I see it, a wife would have been much cheaper than a nanny, and you can't abuse a nanny (or you shouldn't!). I know my grandmother and she loved children. I'm sure she married this man to help those kids.

Meme D. and Pepe were wed on August 3, 1938. Meme D. now had six children to care for, ranging in ages three to ten! She wasn't accustomed to living in a home where they had only outdoor plumbing. Life was challenging for her and little Bev as this was quite an adjustment. In the evenings, Meme D. would rock the youngest of Pepe's kids to sleep as he was the same age as Bev. Baby Bev would put her hands up to be picked up and rocked by her mother, but Meme D. was careful not to show preference to Bev as she was very afraid of Pepe's wrath. He would get very angry if he thought for a second that Meme D. showed Bev favoritism over his children. Meme D. suffered too many beatings to make that mistake, so Bev went to bed most nights without getting rocked by her mother from then on.

Shortly after their wedding, Meme D. had three miscarriages and then gave birth to seven more children! Meme D. now had thirteen children to look after and would have her hands full for many years to come. She had a tight budget to feed all the children and somehow scraped a dinner together every night. Some nights it was a bowl of hamburger soup with bread and butter. Nobody complained as it was always tasty!

The one shining light in little Bev's life was a neighboring lady. Bev would walk by her house on the way home from school and she always had chocolate cake and milk on hand for Bev to snack on. I wonder how much this neighbor knew about their lives. She even offered to adopt Bev as she didn't have children and she knew that Bev was in a tough situation. Of course, Meme D. would never have given Bev up. In fact, it was totally out of the question.

In one of our chats, Mom shared that she had always secretly wished that Meme D. had not married Pepe. She thought it had been an impulsive decision and it wreaked havoc on both their lives. Meme D. must not have been thinking of what was best for little Bev when she married him, and surely had not thought it through. I never had the chance to ask Meme D. if, in fact, she too had wished she hadn't. But she did have seven more kids and I know she adored all her children. So had she not married Pepe D., she would not have had those seven kids.

Being the stepchild was not easy for Mom. She was often told by one or another of her siblings that if she didn't do as she was told, they'd tell Pepe D. and he would throw her out. For a little girl, this was very frightening as she believed them. She was constantly on pins and needles and very afraid of her place in this world. One day while doing their chores, Mom's sister told her to wash the stairs, knowing full well this was her chore. When Mom refused, her sister told her that if she didn't do the chore, she'd tell Pepe D. This is how her sister abused her authority and Mom was forced to do those additional chores from then on.

Life only got harder for Mom once her step-siblings realized her fear. Pepe D. was a mean drinking man and Mom knew better than to test his ire. He beat her often enough, therefore, she did as she was told because she didn't want to give him a reason to beat her more. On one occasion, Pepe D. was very angry with Mom for some offense so she ran out the back door, right through the screen, and kept running until she got to her aunt's house. She stayed there four days and Pepe didn't even notice. She got away with it...that time.

When Mom was about ten years old, Pepe came home from work and dinner was not ready. He was madder than a box of frogs! He usually would sit at the table, drink in hand, until dinner was ready and waited impatiently while Meme got dinner ready while still meeting the needs of thirteen children! On this particular day, he was even more exasperated when dinner wasn't ready on time. Pepe told each of them to grab a chair and to step outside. There sitting on their chairs, all around the apple tree, were Meme D, Mom, her younger brother, and her sister. He had tied them all to the apple tree and held them there at gunpoint. They were all terrified as he was very intoxicated and they feared for their lives. At long last, he fell asleep and a neighbor came over, untied them, and took away the rifle. Meme D. took them inside, gave them each a peanut butter cookie, and said to forget what had just happened! How does one forget that your own father held you captive at gunpoint? I was horrified upon hearing this story. It broke my heart to know my own mother had to live that life. It also explained why we, as children, were never allowed toy guns to play with, not even water pistols. This is peculiar as I, too, had never allowed guns in my home but never really had a reason other than always being told they were dangerous.

Mom's stepbrothers were a whole other dreadful story. When Mom was just five years old, the sexual abuse started. Her older brother initiated it. He would leave his schoolbooks on the table and go upstairs. He'd call on Mom to bring them up to him, then would throw her on the bed and molest her.

Mom shared a double bed with her sister, but we'll never know how her sister didn't know this was going on. Night after night Mom was abused. The abuse, unfortunately, did not end when her older brother moved out – the other brothers got involved too. One of them would give her a piece of mint gum and force her to give him pleasure. It was revolting. She was just a little girl who had no idea what she was doing.

It would be several years before Mom told a single soul of her inner agony and shame. When probed as to why she didn't tell her mother, her only response was that those were hard times and people didn't speak of such things, she didn't dare tell her mother for fear she'd be put out on the street. I seriously doubt that would've happened but this is how she felt.

My mother would never let any of us girls, my sisters and I, stay overnight at our cousins' (the homes of these men), and she would not tell us why. Now we know and I thank her for protecting us in this way.

I often wondered how this abuse affected my mother's opinion of sex and how it played into her married life. I asked her if it had anything to do with my father's wandering ways; would it have made a difference to him if he had known? Would he have been more understanding and perhaps a better husband? Her simple reply was that likely it did. Sex was a painful, shameful thing to her. It never felt right. He was likely picking up on her discomfort and tried to get things done quickly. Sadly, she didn't learn till much later in life that lovemaking is a form of sharing love with your life partner and that it can be a beautiful thing.

Chapter Four

MOM MEETS DAD

May 19, 1951

Dear Diary,

I always wondered how my parents met and today, with very little probing, Mom revealed to me that info! By the way she spoke; you'd think he was this innocent and sweet man. Do you think it's possible that he was back then? Here she was being abused at home, still in her older teenaged years and this man treats her respectfully; she was so defenseless. I think I'd probably be falling in love too if I were as vulnerable as she.

Can you imagine my father had game! It sounds like a very romantic proposal indeed. I'm glad that he didn't lay a hand on Mom, I really respect that. I know that eventually changed but by the way Mom talks, they were genuinely happy and excited to be together. They had their challenges ahead of them but I'm glad they had a nice wedding day and a Niagara Falls honeymoon. Stay tuned, Diary...

It was the May long weekend and Mom and two of her friends were going for a bike ride, a long bike ride. They packed some sandwiches and a jar of juice and headed out on their bikes. Their destination was a friend's farm in Stoney Point, fifteen miles away, home of two of her school chums. Destiny had taken Mom to the family farm, and love was in the making on that fateful day.

It took them all morning to get there but when arrived, her friends greeted them with their friendly smiles. They all had a picnic under a big old shade tree and just relaxed, as they were tired from their trek on the bikes. Mom was introduced to Dad, by his brother and sister, the same friends she had biked all that way there to see. They hit it off right away. She found him handsome and charming; he found her attractive and funny. That sense of humor of hers would later serve her very well in life.

In the weeks following the picnic, you would often find Dad at the basketball games at Belle River District High School even though he wasn't a student, hoping to meet up with Mom. Dad didn't go to high school because his father needed him on the farm. Dad would attend the games with his buddies. These three boys were like the three musketeers! At one of these games, Dad asked Mom to go to the prom. She, of course, said she'd love to, all the while thinking, "What could I possibly wear?"

On the night of the prom, Dad picked Mom up and off they went to dinner first at a local restaurant for spaghetti and meatballs with their friends. Mom was very careful not to spill on her outfit that she had put together herself. She had bought a used red velvet top and a tulle skirt, which she fixed up with matching velvet bows and ribbons. It looked brand new and she was proud of what she had done especially when her friends marveled at her beautiful outfit. Nobody needed to know it was pieced together with a pre-worn skirt and a top bought at the local resale clothing shop. Her objective was to feel pretty and she looked great just like all her friends did!

The prom was a lot of fun and if it had been up to Dad, he would have had his way with Mom, but she didn't let that happen. He had her home at a respectful hour and the evening left him thinking about the future and wanting more.

Mom was sure she had found her escape route to happiness, or so she would believe for years to come. She went to bed that night with sweet dreams for the future. She dreamt of a home filled with children – a home where there was peace and love.

Then on Christmas Eve of 1952, Dad proposed to Mom at Duck Creek Bridge. He pulled over and handed her a ring and proposed marriage, for her to be his wife. She was overjoyed and said yes!

This was the happiest day of her life. She was finally marrying the love of her life! To move out of that house of horrors was just a bonus. She imagined Dad to be the hero who saved her from the big bad world she lived in. Up to this point, he had not laid a finger on her, so she was convinced he was a good man. At this point, Dad had no idea what was going on in Mom's home. He wouldn't learn any of this till much later in life.

On October 17, 1953, they were married in Belle River, Ontario, which was Mom's hometown. They had a morning service which was quite traditional at this time. The family went to the home of Dad's parents in Stoney Point. Meme Q. had a meal arranged at the family farmhouse and had a woman helping her with the meal. They put out a generous bountiful meal and you can be sure many of Meme Q's sweets were freshly baked for this momentous occasion.

They took photos outside as it was a gorgeous fall day. Meme Q. had the most beautiful rose gardens. You could smell them from blocks away! She spent hours in this garden and you could be sure if there was a wedding planned, she'd spend even more time in those gardens.

In the afternoon they went to the convents to visit Dad's two sisters who were religious sisters. Back then the Sisters weren't allowed to go to weddings; they would have had to get special permission just to go home for a visit and especially a wedding. Times were a bit different back then.

For their wedding dinner, they had a reception at the Wellington Tavern in Belle River. The meal cost $5 a plate, a very dear meal at the time. It had all the usual wedding meal items but the one thing that stood out was the cabbage rolls. Mom loved cabbage rolls. It was a dry wedding and there was a swing-era band playing. The first dance was *They Told Us We Were Too Young*. How prophetic that turned out to be as Mom was only eighteen and Dad was twenty.

A midnight snack was served and then the party was over. The day had gone by so quickly! They went to Niagara Falls for a few days on their honeymoon and to start their new lives as man and wife. Like most young newlyweds, they started their married life with hopes and dreams, yet they had no idea what ***life*** had in store for them!

Chapter Five

THE CHILDREN COME MARCHING IN

1954

Dear Diary,

I always wondered about Mom having one child after another, eight in total. She expressed that she never gave it much thought; it was simply what she was meant to do at that given time. They didn't use birth control back then, so the babies came into the world again and again. She said that she just took one day at a time and tried not to plan too much ahead because there was always some kind of trouble, be it bloody noses, someone stepping on a nail, kids fighting, food fights, broken limbs, kids getting hurt at school, chauffeuring one to hockey or another to dance etc. I will keep the "One day at a time" advice in mind in the future. It's great advice that never gets old.

Married life at the beginning was great for Mom and Dad. When they were first wed, they were living on the farm with Meme and Pepe Q. They were loving life and all was going well until the morning when Mom woke up to the smell of bacon frying and she became very ill. Meme Q. knew instantly what this meant: Mom was pregnant.

Over the next twelve years, Mom would have eight kids: four girls and four boys! Mom was a doting mother and had less time for Dad's needs. He was becoming jealous of his own kids. It was immature of my father, but as a couple, Mom and Dad never resolved the issue in a way that satisfied them both. Dad would begrudge his own children getting love and affection from their mother for years, jealous that Mom would spend more time with her kids than him. I guess he overlooked that he was half of the reason he had eight kids!

Dad would even get angry when Mom did laundry for the older boys. Dad thought they should do their own, all the while she was doing Dad's laundry! Kind of ironic I thought when she shared this story with me: Dad, a grown man, had his wife do his laundry but forbade his sons from having his laundry done by their own mother?

Mom would spend many years changing diapers, cloth ones of course, toilet training toddlers, crying when her kids started school, caring for kids when the chickenpox hit one child after another, and tending to skinned knees.

Our household was one of chaos. There were constant fights about whose Barbie was whose and who cut their hair? The boys would wrestle in the living room, having fun till they didn't. There were spats about wanting the red cup, not the yellow one and who got the most milk. Dad had to make a special table that fit all of us at once. It was massive and I wish I knew where that table is today.

The teen years were one nightmare after another for Mom. There were terrible accidents involving three of my siblings. There'd be broken legs, smashed cheekbones, broken pelvises, and concussions. I swear that Mom ran from one hospital to the next! We were driving her mad I do believe.

Having said all that, there were some good times. I remember when I was a little girl, my brother was swinging me around the kitchen while

Mom was preparing dinner. I can still smell the roast cooking in the background, and me smiling and giggling as my brother twirled me to keep me busy while Mom got the meal on the table.

In order to keep things running smoothly in our busy household, we all had chores to do. The boys would take out the garbage and help Dad with any yard work or any building projects he would be on at the time. Dad was always building something...always.

Growing up in our generation meant the girls did the housekeeping chores like dishes, vacuuming, laundry, beds, etc. We were put into teams, two sisters on one team and the other two on the other. One year, I remember that my team sister had to have her appendix out, it was our week for the dishes, and do you know that I had to do them on my own? I was twelve! Let me tell you, there are a lot of dishes with eight kids. The grown-up me reflects back on that and asks, "Why didn't someone step up to help me?"

Because Mom was so busy working in the restaurant and likely taking care of one kid's issue or another, we often helped each other out with the homework. My sister is very gifted in the sewing department and one year for my home-economics project, I was sewing a pair of gauchos. Yes, that's what we called them back then. I brought them home to finish up and my sweet sister not only totally took over and finished those, but fixed my blunders while she was at it. I got a great mark for that project and I don't think I wore them once out in public! They were brown corduroy and very chic. I should've paid better attention though as I still can't sew.

My sister wasn't the only one helping with homework. I have memories of us all sitting at the table after dinner, helping one another with math problems, French quizzes, history, etc. I'd help where I could but I was younger than most of them so I didn't have much to add!

When we weren't at school or doing homework, we were outside playing. My sister (who was closest in age to me) and I often played together as little girls. One of my fondest memories of her is us swinging through the air on our swings and belting out the song

"Stop! In the Name of Love!" To this day, every time I hear that song, I think of her and that period of our lives. It is a lasting memory and considering all that went on in our home, it's a good one! I think that it was rather prophetic on our part to be singing *"Stop! In the Name of Love"* considering what ensued in our lives.

The boys would be playing hockey or baseball outside or they'd be in the ditches fishing for frogs or catfish. I joined them occasionally when they let me but I didn't see the fascination with frogs, snakes, or fish. To me, they were slimy and dirty and I did not want to touch them. Of course, the boys got great fun out of chasing us girls with a toad, or fish. Boys!

As frenzied as it was in our home, I remember it to be a home where we all loved each other most days. Oh sure, there were spats with one another, but when something serious was happening, and that occurred far too often, we all banded together.

I remember when my little brother was just a baby, he had a bad case of bronchitis and stayed in the hospital for a few days. I stood watch by that door waiting for him to get home. I missed him terribly as he was my favorite dolly. He let me feed him, and he pooped for real and giggled like the best dolls ever! That was till he was about seven. He and his friend took apart my Mrs. Beasley doll to see how she could talk. I was so upset that I cried for days. I'm still ticked about that! Mrs. Beasley never spoke again in our home. I was the only one sad about that, you can be sure.

Mom says she regrets many things in her life but having a large family is not one of them. Her children were all worth the trouble and brought her so much joy over the years.

Chapter Six

THE COMING AND GOING OF AUNT SUSIE

Summer 1959

Dear Diary,

I'm still trying to wrap my brain around Aunt Susie moving back in. I know I wasn't abused by my father or brothers as she had been, and perhaps it's not fair to judge, but honestly if you didn't love him, why come back? Why not just say "no"? My take is that it can only be explained by her basement level low self-esteem.

I remember her moving out and I was sad because I loved having her around; yet Mom was in a good mood the day Aunt Susie left. She was happy for her sister, but I think she was happy to have her husband back. Dad on the other hand, WAS NOT happy, and when he's not happy, nobody is! He was very manipulative and would find a way to get her back here in our home where HE wants her. And he did. Whom did he serve by doing that? His wife? NO. Aunt Susie? NO. His children? NO!. HIM and only him!

I always wondered about Aunt Susie moving in. When and why did it happen? Mom conveyed that in the summer of 1959, she found herself pregnant again with her fifth child. She asked her younger sister Susan to come live with the family. The official story was that my aunt would help with the children.

Mom wasn't exactly ecstatic about being pregnant again. It was no wonder she was always pregnant. Dad would come in and summon her to the bedroom with the "come-hither" sign, and she would be expected to drop everything, no matter what she was doing, and perform for him. Was it any wonder she was pregnant again? They never used birth control of any kind until after eight kids!

The truer reason that Aunt Susie came to live with us was that she too was being sexually molested by several of her older brothers. Her four older brothers molested her from the time she was very young, so when she had the chance to move out, she was happy to get out of that turbulent home.

She thought highly of Dad and her older sister, our Mom, so in her mind, it was to be a beautiful thing. She knew she'd be helping with the children, but anything beats getting pawed at every night by one brother or the other.

Mom took Aunt Susie out shopping to get her some new clothes for high school as she was settling in. At first, things went very well and my aunt was happy. The children thrived with the extra help and loved having Aunt Susie around. Mom was getting some much-needed relief as well.

I would not be born for another three years. Eventually, once I was born, I would share a bedroom with Aunt Susie, as she was known to me. We each had our own twin beds and the arrangement seemed to work fine.

Eventually, though, she started getting a visitor at night. My father took up where her brothers left off. To this day, I struggle with this information; he abused Aunt Susie and left us girls alone. Should I be grateful for that? What about overhearing what was going on in the twin bed about an arm's length away? It was simply selfish behavior on my father's part.

It was scary to me; I was just a wee girl. I could hear her protesting, asking him to leave. I was only three years old but somehow I knew something was wrong there. It was dark and I could hear these strange noises.

My earliest memory in life is of me sitting at the kitchen table for breakfast and asking Aunt Susie what all that noise was last night in her bed. I still can see her look up at my father as he was there too, and she leaned in really close to my ear and said, "That's just the monkeys in your dreams." Basically, she was telling a three-year-old that what I heard was all in my mind. Perhaps for the moment, it did get her and Dad off the hook – especially Dad. She made less noise from then on, likely afraid that I'd hear. I suppose that worked perfectly into Dad's agenda.

I was a young woman when I experienced those noises myself and put it all together. It wasn't an enjoyable memory and frankly to this day, I will have the occasional flashback of those nights. It wasn't pleasant then and it's not pleasant now.

When I was about four years old, my aunt got engaged to a young man that she had been dating. Everyone was happy for her except Dad. While we were all out, or so Dad thought, Dad held Aunt Susie by the scruff of her blouse up against the wall and told her she would break up with that man. He told her that he would take care of her and she was not to date ever again. She was crying that she loved that man and Dad said, ***"No, you love me!"*** Aunt Susie stormed off to her bedroom and cried all night. Mom was simply told that Aunt Susie was sad because she had broken up with her fiancé. Another red flag missed by our busy Mom.

I remember as a little girl, when I was around six years old, I was lying in my bottom bunk and thinking, who is my mother? I know I call Bev, Mommy and I call Sue, Aunt Susie, but when Mom is at work,

Aunt Susie cares for us and Dad comes into her room. It was just very confusing for me and likely to my siblings as well. I never once discussed this with anyone until after I was married.

Aunt Susie moved out of our family home somewhere around 1970. All of us kids were in school and it was time for her to move on. Mom was thrilled by the choice: Aunt Susie had a job lined up at a nearby distillery and would live with her widowed mother to help her out more with chores and the rent. It seemed like a great new beginning for her.

Shortly after Aunt Susie moved out, Mom found Dad lying across his bed in the middle of the afternoon, crying. Mom asked him what was wrong. Dad told her that he was sad that Sue had moved out. Truly, he was furious that she had left him behind with the wife and eight kids! When Mom questioned why he was sad, Dad said that he needed her. That should have been a flashing neon sign to Mom, but she took it that he needed her in the restaurant that they owned. She later would tell me that she wanted to believe what he said about needing her, but she really knew the truth of what he meant. She missed yet another huge red flag!

Days later, Dad was out and gone for several hours. When he finally got home, he told Mom that he had "run into" Aunt Susie. He also told Mom that she'd be moving back in. Mom was less than thrilled, to say the least! Mom hadn't even had time to clean out the room! Aunt Susie moved right back into our home and Mom had her favorite apple pie waiting for her as a sign of a warm welcome. Not what I would've done but I don't have Mom's background.

That was to be the first of several attempts on my aunt's part to leave. She was weak and would give in to Dad's demands. He was narcissistic and what he wanted, he got. So even though she was not in love with him, she would move back in. Aunt Susie knew her sister wanted to have her husband to herself but that wasn't enough for Dad.

There would be several more red flags for Mom, but she would look the other way, pretend to not see them, or simply let things slide. Her childhood had instilled a huge fear that she would be put out on the street so she would tolerate the situation, for now.

Aunt Susie stayed until 1992 when Dad finally broke it off with her. He was still married to Mom but was flirting with a twenty-eight-year-old waitress and therefore he fired Aunt Susie. He had a new toy. Aunt Susie was undeniably angry and hurt by this, after all that she gave up in life. She had long passed up on true love, had her tubes tied so that she wouldn't get pregnant by Dad, and abandoned all her young life to a man that was only interested in his needs.

She was dropped like a bad habit, never to have any kind of relationship with Dad ever again. She couldn't help feeling that she was replaced with a newer, fresher model. She was right, she had been.

Just days after their split, Dad was at his beloved Spitfire game, to which he had season tickets. When he came out, all four of his tires had been slashed. There's never been any proof or anyone owing to this vandalism, but I strongly believe Aunt Susie took a little frustration out on some rubber that night! A woman scorned...

Chapter Seven

THE TRAGIC BUS ACCIDENT

December 21, 1966

Dear Diary,

Today I received an article in the mail from the Windsor Star. It was a story about a bus accident that occurred 50 years ago. It happened to be one of my father's trucks that had been involved in the accident. I called Mom and she reminded me of some of the details. I have faint memories of this but I do remember her guiding all of us children, including baby Phil, into a bedroom. She had us all kneel to say a prayer, but I was only four years old, so I was just following the others. I did feel fear, but I didn't know for what, yet I could see it on the older kids' faces, and especially Dad's. I had never seen Dad afraid.

I was glad that I had the nerve to ask Mom. She answered all my questions except for one. I wondered why the newspaper didn't report, 50 years later, how that accident affected the driver's family, or better yet, ours? It was a pivotal moment in all our lives; it was shortly after this incident that Dad started visiting mine and Aunt Susie's room. So many lives changed forever that fateful day.

On Wednesday, December 21, 1966, a new school bus driver was training on the bus route that he needed to learn as he was scheduled to take it over come the New Year. The weather was cold, there was wet snow, and the roads were slippery. The retiring driver warned the new driver to be wary of a specific intersection as it was a busy one. Suddenly, a dump truck skidded to avoid hitting a car. In its attempt to miss that car, the truck side-swiped the bus, and the truck's box and its load of sand started to tip. The sand smashed the bus's windows and its roof, dumping the sand into the bus carrying thirty young children. Few of the children would get off that bus unharmed.

The first people on the scene clawed at the sand with their bare hands, turning up a portion of a hand or a leg connected to screeching children. They even uncovered books and lunch pails. The scene was one of chaos; there were ear-piercing sirens of all types and people trying to find their children. You could feel the hysteria in the air.

Later these rescuers would report children screaming and crying that they were suffocating in the mounds of sand. The scene was one of pandemonium; two fire departments, two police departments, and two ambulance services were all trying to help thirty little kids. There was a welder on his way home from work. Someone handed him a torch and while they jacked the bus up, he went under it to cut holes in the floor of the bus, ultimately freeing the children. Sadly, while this welder was working away, he could hear the cries of one child who later died before he could free him. This was harder for him to accept than the danger he was facing working with a torch only six inches away from the gas tank.

One mother of a Grade 1 student at the local public school was driving two car lengths behind the bus. As she neared the scene, she realized it was her daughter's bus and became frantic when she saw the truck and its load dumped into the bus. She stopped her car, got out, and started running when she saw her little girl wandering around the bus, likely suffering from shock. Her mother threw her into the car and drove straight to the hospital where her daughter remained overnight for observation. Ultimately, she suffered very few physical wounds – only a small number of cuts to her face. Thank the good Lord for looking out for this child.

Another young lady was waiting for her sister to arrive on the bus. She saw the bus sitting at the intersection which was the next stop for her little sister. When she realized the bus had been hit, she ran out and jumped aboard the bus's emergency door at the back of the bus, calling out to her little sister whose legs were pinned by the seat ahead of her. Someone came and cut the legs of the seat away and big sister carried her little sister off that horrifying bus. The little girl sat in her big sister's arms at the accident scene until paramedics had a look at her. Miraculously she was not hurt and went home with her sister. This big sister had been her little sister's caregiver since their mother's recent death. When their father arrived home early from work, all the little one could say was "I don't hurt." He knew they were one of the lucky families because already, three families from this street had lost children that day.

A good Samaritan was on his way home from work when he witnessed the accident. He jumped on the bus to see how he could help when he spotted another little girl pinned by the seat ahead of her. He sat crouched for over an hour with this frightened little girl in his arms. He comforted her while others struggled to free her pinned legs. She hardly spoke other than to say that her legs hurt. She also said she had a brother on the bus. She was to be the last victim removed from the bus. Both of her legs were broken but she survived the ordeal. Her brother had been one of the first children to get off the bus. He had been sitting behind the driver and managed to get out as soon as the bus was hit.

In all, eight children died and sixteen were injured. The children ranged in ages six to nine. The children were all pupils of a local public school in Sandwich South Township.

At the very time of the accident, Dad, the owner of the truck that hit the bus, was Christmas shopping in Tilbury. He was at a jewelry store picking out a little something for Mom, the mother of his eight kids. He stopped in next door at his insurance agent to wish him a Merry Christmas. This is where and when he heard of the accident. Dad's lawyer had called the insurance agent and told him to tell Dad to get home and he'd meet him there. Dad wanted very badly to go help at the accident scene but was advised against this by his lawyer, who was afraid Dad would be lynched because the parents were angry, to say the least.

Once home, Dad had Mom take all eight of us children into one bedroom and we were told to keep quiet. Oddly enough, we did stay quiet. Mom and all of us children knelt around the bed and prayed to God for the speedy recovery of children injured in the accident. At the time, I was only four, so I didn't understand what was happening but somehow I knew this was big and just followed the lead of my older siblings.

Dad and his lawyer sat in the kitchen for an hour and every once in a while, I'd hear a few of Dad's French curses come out of his mouth. They finally went out to the car to finish their conversation where they wouldn't be heard by us. Dad sold the trucking business that night to a friend and neighbor because Dad knew that he'd not be able to get insurance or run a trucking business again after this horrific accident... nor did he want to.

The driver was charged with dangerous driving and was taken into custody at the accident scene. His life from that moment forward was changed for the rest of his life.

The driver of the car that caused the truck to skid was never found. There was no information regarding him in any of the newspaper articles. To this day, we still have problems with people who cause accidents and just drive away. The good news is that there are cameras or eyes everywhere now so drive safely people, please.

The truck driver's family, wife, and sons would stay with our family for days to come. They were with us on Christmas Eve where we celebrated "reveillon" early. Normally you'd stay up late, go to Midnight Mass, eat the traditional tourtière, and get to bed at a very late time. This year we only had the tourtiere for dinner, but no reveillon. The children were there when we woke Christmas morning after Santa had come. Those children were also quite young, so they didn't understand the depth of what was happening. For that, we can all be grateful. In cases like this, ignorance is bliss.

There were no Christmas lights or dazzling displays this year for our family. It was a time of sadness and it seemed the whole area was mourning, which was understandable after such a horrific accident and numerous loss of lives.

What we didn't expect on Christmas morning was the black wreath someone had hung on our front door. There was a banner on it that read, "Your eight kids are next." This was incredibly upsetting for my parents, especially Mom; she needed to be consoled. Her children were everything to her, and now she was very concerned for our safety.

In spite of the perceived danger, Mom and Dad decided to go to church regardless of the threat and pray for the families of the eight children who died in the accident. Mom and Dad tried not to think of the irony – they were sitting in church with their eight young children while praying for the families who had lost a total of eight children who wouldn't be in church with their families on this day or ever again.

The press was assuming details and blaming the driver before all facts were even known and the public was in an uproar. It was a terrible situation to say the very least but surely the press or public could not possibly believe that the driver set out that morning thinking he'd go out and cause an accident that would kill eight children. He was devastated. His life changed forever as soon as that car cut him off and he swerved to miss him.

Life for Mom and Dad and our family had been very good until this accident but was about to change in an immense way. This is when Dad started to confide in Aunt Susie late at night when Mom was tired and finally in bed after chasing and doing things for eight kids all day. The tragedy would change the course of our lives for years to come.

In the months and years that followed there would be court cases, insurance claims to settle, and grief to be dealt with. Dad would sit up until the wee hours and talk it out with Aunt Susie. She had a great ear for listening and was very good at making him feel better. It didn't much time for things to turn into a relationship and before long, Dad and Aunt Susie were entangled in a mess that would last a very long time.

The final court case involved a couple who lost their only child, a girl. His wife was suffering a broken heart because of their daughter's death. The case was dragged out the longest and the one that my father was most concerned about. This family was seeking a very large settlement.

I was young but I remember my father coming home from court as we were all waiting for him. My mother jumped up when he walked in, and Dad said the case had been dropped by the man. This very brave father said that all the money in the world would not bring back his wife or child and he didn't want to ruin our family too. I had never seen my father show any sign of affection to my mother, ever in my life, until that moment. All eight of us just stood there and watched Dad kiss Mom and they both had tears of joy on their faces. It was one of those happy but sad moments.

I want to express to the families of those eight children who died that fateful day: I am so incredibly sorry this happened. My heart goes out to you and I want you to know that we've thought of you and prayed for you many times over the years. My hope for you and your families is peace, healing, and love.

Chapter Eight

THE RESTAURANT YEARS

1967

Dear Diary,

OH MY GOD, can you imagine Diary if your husband bought a restaurant without even discussing it with you? I mean, come on! I was only four at the time, so I don't remember a lot of the arguments, but I do remember a lot of commotion! The big kids, would shoo us little ones off to a different room or outside if Mom and Dad started arguing. All I can say is it wouldn't fly in my household, but I have Mom to thank for that. Despite her constant compliance to Dad, I told myself I'd never be subservient to my husband when I grew up. Good grief, how does a man get away with this crap? How can Mom be so naïve? Seriously, why didn't my Aunt speak up? I mean it was still early in the making, relatively, and it would've changed the course of our lives had she or someone said something! I am glad though that Dad is taking my brother on a trip; I'm sure Mom thought he'd be in Dad's room and that would keep Aunt Susie out, boy o boy Diary...

In the spring of 1967, Dad was still out of work as he had sold the trucking company to his neighbor after the bus accident. He didn't regret that decision for a moment until one day when he was driving through town and saw one of the trucks parked in front of the Stoney Point Tavern. He locked on his brakes and went inside.

There he found that same friend sitting on a bar stool having a beer. Dad told him to go and move the truck because he was concerned that those trucks still had his name on them and he had a case before the courts. If someone should see "his" trucks in front of a tavern, they'd jump to the conclusion that his drivers were drunks.

The owner of the establishment asked Dad to stop chasing his customers off unless Dad owned the place, then he could tell people to get out. Dad asked if the place was for sale. The owner's reply was that anything is for sale. Dad made a deal with the owner right then and there! He then headed to his lawyers to seal the deal to buy a restaurant. He had never in his life worked in a restaurant or owned one. He didn't know the first thing about running this kind of establishment. To say Dad was impulsive would be a colossal understatement!

Not only did he do this without consulting his wife, but he had the lawyers explain it all to her, including the fact that Mom would be working in the restaurant every day to help and if it were to work out, she'd be a big part of that. She thought Dad was a coward but decided to help because it's who she was. She thought it her responsibility to support all of her husband's decisions, no matter how irrational they were!

Mom was concerned that she still had eight kids to nurture while working at the restaurant but nevertheless, she was expected to work as hard as anybody else. No, that's wrong...she was expected to work ***harder*** than anyone else.

That August, our family moved into the apartment above the restaurant and with some renovations, Mom and Dad made it a very comfortable home for the family. There were seven bedrooms and one bathroom.

Mom and Dad had the room at the end of the hallway. The other rooms were all split up between the kids. I again shared a room with Aunt Susie. It ended up being the closest to the kitchen and living room but the farthest from Mom and Dad's.

There was a family meeting with the kids to explain that times were tough. and they needed to be careful about not wasting and not to ask for any new things. The first years proved to be very tight financially for the family. I remember them saying we had to scrimp on things, even toilet paper. We were expected to use only four sheets of toilet paper when we used the facilities! That took much explaining for some of us! For some reason this is the detail that I remember from the meeting the most – it had hit a nerve with a few of the kids for sure.

At first, the Stoney Point Tavern (SPT) was all about beer and chips. Then Mom started making sandwiches at lunchtime, and in the winter she'd make a pot of soup which would sell out during lunchtime, as well. Then Dad added a grill and a fryer to her tiny kitchen and put burgers, fries, and fish on the menu. SPT was becoming more popular and slowly the business grew. Mom was working later and later.

Sadly, my little brother and I also sat and waited for Mom to come upstairs to be with us. For the older kids, Mom working hard meant more freedom; time to run the streets! For us little ones, it meant loneliness, wanting for our Mommy.

Eventually on Saturday nights, Dad started adding entertainment in the form of bands so that when people came for dinner, they'd stay for the entertainment. My little brother and I, the two youngest children, would sit at night in the stairway to the apartment, peeking in the restaurant to watch the bands. We loved to watch the crowd dancing, laughing, and the band singing their hearts out! We also knew come Sunday morning, we would be allowed downstairs to pick up all the change that fell out of the men's pockets. We'd get to keep what we found and bought a lot of candy with that change! A bag full of penny candy would, at most, cost us twenty-five cents! I have the fillings to prove it too.

Adding the entertainment meant the riffraff would come out too. In particular, one group who came in from Leamington was unhappy that we had a black man singing on our stage. He was a wonderful singer and to us, it was a no-brainer. In fact, I don't know if it ever occurred to my parents not to have him on stage. But the gang that opposed it were a rough bunch and it caused quite a brawl! Our dog Gus, a big black Bouvier, was sent to chase them off the property but unfortunately, the gang was armed with pipes. Gus had seen his last battle and went off to a "farm" to live out his life, or so we were told. Dad's backup plan was to call on his army, which consisted of my older brother, his local pals, Dad's regulars, our uncles, anybody that we could use to defend the Stoney Point Tavern and its guests. It was quite the melee. As kids, we watched in horror from our relative safety, the upstairs windows. We saw Mom throw a cast iron fry pan at some dude from the kitchen door, and she nailed him! "That's my mom!" I shouted out. There were some minor wounds but for the most part, as far as I know, they were all weary but without major injuries.

Then on another night altogether, while most of us were sleeping, Dad heard some noise down in the restaurant. It was closed and there should be no noise. As he went to check it out, he grabbed one of the boys' many hockey sticks dragging at the top of the stairs. He walked in and there was a man trying to break open the cash box on the shuffleboard. In the dark, Dad with his hockey stick pointed straight at the guy and shouted, ***"Stop or I'll shoot!"*** The man bolted for the door, jumped in his car, and drove off with his head down. As he sped away, Dad whacked the car with the hockey stick and the car veered across the road, missed the school by inches, went right through the school fence, drove clear across the schoolyard, and then drove through the other fence! It was the talk of the town for weeks, and someone hung the hockey stick on the wall of the restaurant as a reminder of Dad's heroism. If anything, my dad was a fearless man.

These types of incidents were becoming more and more frequent, so Dad decided to remove the bar from the restaurant.

The Stoney Point Tavern was turning out to be very popular, so much so that Dad had to build one addition and then another. He did remove the bar, much to the chagrin of the local beer drinkers, but Dad had to think of the business he could grow rather than the little business he would lose. His theory was that if his dining customers came in to find drinkers at the bar, they'd feel less welcome. To that point he was right. Business grew tremendously after he built the new kitchen, removed all the shuffleboards, pinball machines, and arcade-type games, and redecorated.

Mom was working harder than ever and we, her children, would look out the window on a Saturday night to see how long the lineup was to get into the restaurant. We would then guess how long she'd be gone based on the length of the line. This was our new normal. SPT was the "it" spot for Saturday dinner, and in the summer with the cottage population, it was even crazier!

The Broasted Chicken and seafood were a huge hit and having an "all you can eat soup and salad bar" were a bonus to the guests. No one ever went home hungry from the Stoney Point Tavern. They offered a land and sea platter that included shrimp, crab, ribs, chicken, scallops, perch, and frog legs which were also served with vegetables and potatoes. It was a dinner for two and rarely did it get finished as it also included soup and salad bar. The customers loved it, and once word got out, it got even busier! People were coming from far and wide to eat at the Stoney Point Tavern.

Were you ever a guest? I'd love to hear the stories of your experiences at the SPT!

In the summer of 1967, Dad packed the car so that he and my brother could go on a fishing trip. Or so my brother was told. They also had two other passengers tagging along: Mom's sisters, Aunt Susie and another aunt of mine. Mom did not want Aunt Susie to go along, but Dad made her feel bad by saying, "How can you take this opportunity away from her?"

My brother found it rather odd at the time that his aunts were there and not his mom, but he was just happy to be going on a road trip with his dad and getting away from the rest of the children. As a child, he was allergic to just about every food that God put on this earth and it did a number on his gastrointestinal system. He forever had gas or worse. No sooner had they hit the highway heading east when his stomach started churning. He had gas so bad and the car reeked horribly of his flatulence. Dad made it to the service center in Dutton, pulled in, and sent him to the bathroom. He told him not to return until he had taken care of his business. That part of the trip still to this day makes my brother smile.

Well, they got back on the road and Dad broke the news to him – they were ***not*** going fishing, and instead, they were going to Montreal to the Expo. You must understand that Expo 67 was also the celebration of Canada's Confederation in 1867. It was studied in school all year; everyone drew pictures and it was my brother's earliest recollections of political parties and government. They arrived in Montreal, got to their hotel on St. Anne Blvd, and prepared for the three-day stay. Dad was in one room, while the two aunts and my brother were in the other room. My brother found this arrangement strange, however, he was glad to be in Montreal and it was absolutely his very first trip away from home. The next three days were kind of a blur and they covered every exhibit at Expo, most of which were just amazing for a kid from Pointe-aux-Roches. The Japanese display was fabulous, and at the German display, he participated in a Volkswagen commercial explaining how double joint axles worked. People were surprised that a 13-year-old kid knew all of this! At the Russian exhibit, they featured huge sturgeons. Dad decided to grab one by the tail and it went nuts thrashing about. This was the most fun, perhaps the only fun my brother ever had with Dad. Dad even bought him some candy popcorn, which he considered good but not quite as good as his Mom's.

Although my brother was grateful for the trip and had a fabulous time, something still did not seem right without Mom being there, while her two sisters were. To this day, some fifty-two years later, my brother still questions the whole scenario and whether there was something he could have done differently, even though he was just a kid.

It ceases to amaze me that a man can go away with his two sisters-in-law and his son and not one adult questioned it? Today, it would be all over social media. Your life is an open book now. I'm not sure that's any better but perhaps we can all endeavor towards a happy medium, that if we witness unseemly behavior by our relatives or friends, we take them aside privately and discuss it with them. If it continues, you may need to make an uncomfortable decision and speak with your sister/mother/brother, etc.

I whole heartily believe that many people knew of my father's goings-on, but none acted on it to him, to my knowledge. Mom says nobody approached her ever regarding Dad until they had split up.

During my research, I have heard many people say they talked to their friends or spouses about it but never talked to Dad or Mom. Even an anonymous letter may have helped with this situation. So if you're facing circumstances like this today, think of possibly writing a letter to your friend, not because you want to be mean-spirited but because you want to stop further damage. At the very least it will start a conversation for the couple, an interesting one at that! I think that's better than gossiping – that has never helped anyone out.

Chapter Nine

LIFE WITH TEENAGERS IN THE 1970s

Dear Diary,

My goodness, it's no wonder Dad gets away with what he does. Mom is so busy caring for 8 kids, most of us are teenagers, she's running a very busy kitchen in our family restaurant and trying to keep our household functioning! The poor woman is beyond exhausted as she gets zero help from Dad as he says he's busy managing the restaurant. I'm sure I'll have more to write soon Diary...

The seventies were a blur for Mom. She had to deal with school issues, graduations, first communions, and confirmations. There were four weddings, at least three of her kids were involved in major car accidents, and by the close of the seventies, all eight of her kids would be going through the teenage years. Imagine the hormones?

On a cold February afternoon in 1973, my brother had been in a very bad car accident. There was a snowstorm, he was headed home for lunch, and the roads were icy. He slid off the road and hit a tree head-on. You could see the shape of the tree in the front of his car! He shattered his cheekbone among other injuries, but to me this was devastating. I was worried sick about him. When he got home from the hospital, I happened to be in the washroom. As I was walking out, he was walking in the door. His swollen black and blue face was unrecognizable.

In the summer of 1975, another brother was in a hockey camp in St. Clair Beach. He and a bunch of his hockey buddies were outside on a break, all sitting on some fella's car when he came out and said he was just moving his car to a different spot. Well, that guy took them on a joy ride in the parking lot, while the boys clung to the car. Three boys left camp that day in an ambulance! Just one more grey hair for Mom.

On a cold fall day in 1975, I was on my way home from school. I stopped for the mail and I talked with the lady who ran the post office, something I usually did. It was her who told me, on this day, that another one of my brothers had been in a terrible car accident. She didn't have all the details but knew it was serious. Imagine telling a child this?

It turns out that my brother took the bend a bit too fast and rolled his Pinto. That's right, a Pinto. Luckily, it did not explode. He did break his leg though and when he got home from the hospital, I waited on him hand and foot. I was thirteen and adored my brother. The thought that he could have died shook me to the core. I would have done anything for my brother and would to this day.

Two weeks later he was the best man at another of our brother's wedding and made his way down the aisle on crutches. They had to specially make his tuxedo pants, he wore a special sock on his foot, and he had a wheelchair for the party.

The following year was my sister's turn to get married. I remember a lot of planning and discussions going on at this time but the thing that sticks in my craw was my dress! I was fourteen and was to stand in her wedding with her fiancé's younger sister. The bridal party all went shopping for our dresses, ordered them, and two months later when they finally arrived, my dress turned out to be too small around the bust area. I had developed a lot in two months. I was fourteen and still growing. There was a bit of commotion about it at first, but then we realized one of the other bridesmaid's dresses was too big, so we switched and all was well. I did bust out of the dress a bit, but I don't remember anybody making comments to me about it. The wedding went on as planned. It was beautiful and they're still married today!

Another of my sisters would get married only six months later. Imagine three large weddings to plan and pay for in exactly one year. I also stood in this wedding. Luckily I had no dress issues and as far as I know, all went well with that wedding too. They also are still married to this day!

The next summer, still another sister gave us quite a fright when she too was in a car accident. She and two friends naively got in a car for a drive with two strange young men, who were from out-of-town. They went speeding around the Comartin bend, an infamous bend in the road in Stoney Point, which they took far too fast. They rolled their car, a Gremlin, known for its terrible handling on the road. My sister and her friends were thrown around like rag dolls as they had not been wearing seat belts. One friend fared the worst with a broken back, arms, and legs. My sister, who was sitting in the middle, flew between the bucket seats and crashed into the gear shift, fracturing her pelvis. She also broke her front teeth when she hit the dashboard. The other friend somehow was left unhurt and drove with my parents to the hospital. She bore the brunt of my father's panic as he yelled at her all the way to the hospital in Windsor, while they followed the ambulance.

The year 1978 would bring another wedding. My brother and his fiancée wed in October of that year, where I stood as a junior bridesmaid once again. It would be my first date with my sweetie! Life was just getting started for me.

My younger brother was a funny little boy and was a people pleaser from the get-go. He did almost anything we asked of him which I'm certain came in handy many times in life. I'm pretty sure he even took up the game of hockey to please Dad. When he was just fourteen, Dad was so positive that my brother would follow in our cousin's footsteps to the NHL that Dad moved him to Windsor to live with his brother and sister-in-law not long after they were married.

He did get scouted in Windsor and made it to Junior A for St. Michael's in Toronto. Living in Toronto was fun for a while but eventually, he got lonely and wanted to come home. He sadly gave the sport up competitively although he still plays hockey today and I'm glad he does because he's a natural and it's fabulous exercise, not to mention a stress reliever. We can all use a stress reliever in today's world.

Those 70s were surely a stressful time for Mom. When we chatted about them often, she expressed again that she simply took life one day at a time back then, so as to not feel overwhelmed. She said she'd pray to God for whatever the day's issue was and then it was often over and done in no time.

Back then I didn't give much thought to Mom's feelings or all of her stresses. She was so very strong. She just toiled away in that hot kitchen while dealing with one fire after another.

If life is stressing you out, maybe take a page from Mom's playbook. Take a deep breath, work on today's issues, and give your worries to God. One day at a time worked for her...maybe it will work for you too.

Part Two

LOVE, MARRIAGE, BETRAYALS, ADVENTURE

Chapter Ten

OUR BABY GIRL ARRIVES – AUGUST 7, 1980

August 7, 1980

Dear Diary,

Dear God, at the birthing classes they said the contractions would feel like gas pains. Gas pains my ass! This feels as if there's a semi-truck rolling around inside my gut, what the Hell? OMG there's another ... breathe, breathe. OK, I think it's time to call Denis, he'll help me through this. Thank the Lord, he's on his way, I'm not sure I can do this without him. Wish me luck because I don't know what I'm doing and, as everyone says, you can't back out now! OK God, I promise, if you help me get this semi out of me and soon I will be a good mother, I will do whatever it takes to make sure he or she has whatever it is they need. To distract myself I day-dream that if he ever asks me to marry him, I'll say yes! I feel as if I've known him all my life. I know he's a good man, I know he'll be a good father to our wee baby. Also, I like the name Bacon, I mean who doesn't love bacon?

October 1, 1981

Dear Diary,

Well Diary, this is the BIG news, we are moving to Toronto. I am terrified, I mean shitless. I know no one there, we have very little money but I don't think that's a problem really, I'll work. The problem is it's a big city mean HUGE, I'm putting on a brave face for Denis but I am afraid. Who am I kidding, we're probably gonna kill it! I'm outta here!

October 1, 1991

Dear Diary,

Oh My! Shit has officially hit the fan. If this wasn't my family that is happening to, I'd say that our family was some kind of soap opera, I think I'd name it "As My Stomach Turns". I mean Mom finally asked for the truth and I knew I'd regret not telling her, but here I am. Now we got people sitting in corn fields spying on their father, we got our mother jumping curbs after her unfaithful husband, I mean if this isn't the makings of a soap opera, at least make into a book. Huh fat chance. I'm told you need a BA at least to write a book. Pfft screw that, I'll write that book if I want to!

The day that our first baby was born was a hot and muggy one – a typical summer day in Stoney Point, especially when you live on a lake.

I asked my Mom to French braid my hair to keep me cool. She often had done this when I was a little girl and I don't know how I knew that I'd need my hair back that night, but somehow, I did. The contractions started late afternoon and were far apart. Denis was at a friend's place that night, but he had said to call if I thought I'd need to go to the hospital. I called him at 7 p.m. and asked him to come over, which he did right away. I was timing the contractions as I had learned in the birthing classes that we'd attended together, and they were getting closer.

Around 10 p.m. we decided to head to the hospital in Mom's red Cougar as it was a smoother ride than Denis's Toyota. I was really hoping my water wouldn't break all over the white interior!

At the hospital, we were greeted by my cousin who was the labor and delivery nurse on duty. My mother has never admitted it to me, but I do suspect she called my cousin to let her know I was on my way. Either that or fate was working on my side as she was just an incredible nurse. She helped me through all the breathing, and Denis's breathing too! He was very helpful and strong and remained there the whole time. He never left my side, not even for a second. At 2:50 a.m. our little girl was born into this world of ours and she's brought joy and happiness into our lives ever since. I was also very grateful for that BBQ steak mom had rustled up for dinner as I ended up needing the strength for labor! Who knew how tiring that'd be?

When our daughter first arrived, we lived with my parents at their home on the lake in Stoney Point. This was a grand arrangement initially and I will always be grateful for their help but eventually, we needed to have our own home. We moved into a little cottage on the lake and together we were a happy family. We didn't need a big house full of fancy things to be happy, we just needed each other.

Our daughter was an adorable little toddler. She was quiet and happy to play all on her own or with her cousins. They would spend hours playing house or school. They were two peas in a pod and still are today. She loved her books and would sit at her little desk pretending to read stories or do homework while her Papa was doing his own homework. Somehow this little girl knew we had a hard-enough life and gave us no trouble at all.

Mom was being supportive by bringing over care packages which might include veggies, breads, pastas, fruit, etc. Pretty much anything she had in the house was put into these packages! I know it was her way of helping and we appreciated the food, there was no doubt. She kept a close eye on us as I think she still worried about our child but we got by just fine. We did surprisingly well considering we were still teenagers.

Dad didn't believe in helping out his kids. His theory was that once you left the nest, fly, fly little birds! On one occasion when we first moved out and were still figuring out how to get from paycheck to the next paycheck, we were low on funds for our rent. I went to Dad to borrow $100. He gave me a long lecture about not wasting, saving your money, on and on. After what seemed like hours, but I'm sure it was minutes, he pulled a wad of bills out of his pocket, counted off $100, reminded me that payday was on Thursday, and he expected to be reimbursed then. I did pay him back and I never asked again!

We were getting in our groove and life was moving at a quick clip. Finally, Denis asked me to marry him! I thought he'd never ask! All of her life, a girl dreams of a man getting down on his knees, maybe with a bouquet in his arms, and perhaps a diamond so big it blinds you when he opens that little box. Or possibly he'll rent a plane and have a banner pulled behind it reading "Marry me Anne-Marie" ...then fifty different Anne-Maries are calling their guys! Okay, maybe that's getting carried away.

But for me, my proposal came on a night when Denis and I were helping my sister. Her husband was out of town although she'd recently had gall-bladder surgery and had a two-year-old son plus their newborn little girl.

That evening after the babies and their mom were tucked in bed, Denis asked me to marry him! I thought at first he was joking or playing with me but when I realized he was serious, of course, I said yes! There were no flowers or fancy ring, but none of that mattered to me. I knew I wanted to spend the rest of my life with this man and was thrilled with finally being asked.

When I look back on that moment, I didn't think much about the proposal and its timing, as it wasn't really that romantic at all. But upon reflection, after helping with the kids all night, I think he got a taste of what family is and wanted to be sure he owned up to his responsibilities. I will always be grateful to Denis for his support while I was pregnant. He never once wavered or threatened to leave me, not even when the hormones got crazy! And believe me, they did.

So, we had a wedding to plan now. I spoke with Mom and she got the ball rolling. We wanted a small wedding, something intimate. But with big families like ours, that was not going to be easy to pull off. Mom took care of most of the arrangements, from flowers to food. Denis and I planned for a photographer and to this day I am glad we afforded the expense. My dress was created by my mother's seamstress and it was beautiful in its simplicity. She delivered what I had asked of her. My sister was my maid of honor and her husband was the best man. We kept it as simple as possible.

One of the details I was not crazy about was the date. We decided on October 27, 1980, which was a Monday. The reason we had to get married on a Monday was that my father did not want to close the restaurant on a Saturday or even a Friday as it would be too much lost revenue. Since he was footing the bill for most of the expenses, I did not feel I had a say in this one, so we went with it.

On Sunday night, the night before our wedding, my father and my brothers tore up the very large dining room floor of the restaurant so that they could lay a new carpet. My husband-to-be spent his last single night working like a slave for my father.

We decided on a church wedding here in our village of Stoney Point, Ontario. We wanted to make our promises of love and our vows to honor one another before God, our families and friends. We wanted to show everyone that even though we were young, we were committed for the long haul. I'm happy to report that we have been committed for thirty-nine years and counting!

After the traditional ceremony, the immediate family proceeded to have the wedding dinner at our favorite restaurant in Windsor, where we had eaten almost weekly while dating. The guests, our siblings, their spouses, as well as parents and grandparents all had the choice of what they'd like for dinner. A special menu had been printed out and the guests had the choice of chicken, veal, beef, or fish. Of course, we had cakes and cookies too!

From there the reception party moved to my parents' place at the lake in Stoney Point. It was an ideal location as the house was large and people could mingle easily. We had approximately 125 people present, and you would never have known it as they were spread out all through the house. Around 9 p.m. another meal was put out by my parents. It was unreal and I had no idea they were doing it. They served shrimp and crab, dips, meats, cheeses, and nibbles of all kinds. There was drinking and dancing happening all over the house. It was a wonderful night and we were grateful to our parents for the party they put on for us.

We left our precious baby, who was only two months old, with my aunt to be cared for while we took a short honeymoon to London, Ontario. We stayed at a little hotel near the airport strip, but it's no longer there. I remember we went out to dinner that night and I ordered a "pink lady" because I thought it sounded so grown-up. It tasted horrid but I drank it anyway. We had very little money and I wasn't about to waste it. We had booked for three nights but could barely stay for two as we missed our little pumpkin so much. We headed home early, picked her up, and spent the rest of our time off quietly at home. I never regretted that decision as it was where we needed to be at the time. Little did I know it would be twenty years later before we had a real honeymoon.

It turned out that our baby brought luck to my aunt's crib. They had been on a waiting list for years to adopt, with no calls whatsoever. Our little girl christened that crib while we were on our honeymoon and just days later, they got a call that a baby boy waiting to be loved by them. Of course, it's possible that it was all a coincidence. That little boy was about to enter a very big family.

A couple of months after we were married, during a chilly fall day, dinner was being prepared in my tiny kitchen at the cottage when the phone rang. It was my sister who lived in the same town as me. She was calling to invite me to a family meeting at her place that evening with just the siblings, but no parents. She wanted to know if I could come and I said, "Of course, family matters are always of importance to me." It seemed the topic was going to be one we had never discussed before with each other or anyone else for that matter: Dad and his promiscuity. Did anyone at this meeting believe that Dad was having an affair with Aunt Susie?

Nobody could have predicted the storm of information that would flow that evening. Apparently, most of us had experiences where we caught Dad in compromising situations and we had all been warned not to tell Mom or anyone else. Except for me, neither Dad nor Aunt Susie knew what I knew about them.

We took turns telling our stories. My sister went first. When she was nine years old, she had been playing with her dolls behind the sofa, a favorite hiding place to get some quiet in our chaotic home. Suddenly out of nowhere, she heard tires screeching, Dad and Aunt Susie came into the house. Dad was shouting, which he always did when he was angry. My sister was frightened and sunk lower behind the sofa. Little did she know that another sister was hiding behind a chair in the kitchen, witnessing the very same scene. Dad was furious, as Aunt Susie had become engaged the night before and she had the nerve to be happy! He held Aunt Susie against the wall by the scruff of her blouse and told her she must break up with him right away. She was hysterically crying and very upset. She didn't want to break it off; she loved him very much she proclaimed. Dad told her he'd take care of her and that he loved her, not this man. Aunt Susie relented and agreed to break it off with her beloved fiancé. I can't help but wonder how life would have been different for her, my mother, and all of us children had she held her ground and married the man she really loved.

That day, the fiancé showed up in a brand new red convertible with an armful of red roses. He was chased away by Dad. Aunt Susie was in her room crying as we'd never heard before. Mom thought Aunt Susie was upset because they broke off their engagement.

Another sister's story told us a different tale. She was five years old and Mom was at the hospital having just given birth to me. My sister was looking for Aunt Susie and eventually found her. At this same time, Dad had been doing renovations as child number seven (me) was on the way and we needed more space. The bathroom door had no knob, so there was a big hole in the door where normally there'd be a knob. Aunt Susie was having a bath, and being a five-year-old, my sister was looking through the hole to see if that was actually Aunt Susie in the bathroom. She heard giggling and upon peeking, she saw Dad and Aunt Susie in the tub together. She was confused by this sight yet didn't talk to anybody about it until this very night.

Once my brother was looking for Dad and was told he was in his office at the restaurant. My brother went to the office and found the door was locked, so he knocked. There was no answer, but he could hear noises inside. A few minutes later, my father and Aunt Susie came walking out of the office together. They weren't very subtle and my brother knew exactly what had been going on.

I told my story and my siblings were astonished. I shared a room with Aunt Susie when I was very little. We had separate twin beds in a fairly small room; small enough that I could almost touch her hand if she reached out to touch mine from her bed. I remember waking up one night when I was three years old. It was dark and I could hear some noises in the bed next to me. I thought someone was hurting my dear Aunt Susie. I fell back to sleep and didn't think of it again until morning when I was having my cereal prepared by Aunt Susie, as I called her. I asked her what that noise was the night before and she said, "Oh, it's only the monkeys in your dreams." To this day I remember that morning vividly. I was having puffed rice with milk and a glass of orange juice, as were most of my siblings who were right there at my side. I never gave that night another thought until this meeting and this very evening. I was an adult woman now and knew exactly what those noises meant.

After everyone had their say and shared their stories, it was unanimously decided that very likely dad was still having an affair with Aunt Susie. After an extremely heated debate, it was settled that we were not to tell Mom the truth unless she asked us. Some of those present believed that Mom likely knew and if she wanted a change, she'd do it. Little did I know it would be another twelve years before she asked me about Dad having an affair.

That night I went to bed with a heavy heart as that evening we made a decision that could affect all our lives. Did we make the right choice? Did Mom have a right to know? Did we have the right to withhold this information from her? Was it really best for Mom? I hoped I wouldn't live to regret this. I wish my older siblings would hear me when I speak. They think I'm just a child. Maybe in their eyes, I am.

Chapter Eleven

THE TORONTO YEARS – 1981 TO 1985

Dear Diary,

Well, we finally made it! Good grief, what a trek it was! Our rental truck broke down on the 401, I guess the radiator was leaking so we had to stop and refill it three times along the way! Denis took my spaghetti container, dumped it and used ditch water to fill the rad, yes, three times! Oh my, I thought we'd never get here. Now that we are, the place is filthy; I have never seen such dirt! It'll take me days to clean it!

Denis, our little girl, and I moved to Toronto on October 1, 1981. He was twenty, I was nineteen, and we had a one-year-old. Denis was enrolled to go to the technology institute. We packed all our meager belongings into a rental van, had our first and last month's rent cheques ready, had $75 in the bank, and then hit the 401 eastbound! We thought we had the world by the tail and given that we thought it, maybe we did.

We had an apartment rented out that we had found earlier in the summer. We were excited about starting fresh. We had no friends or family in Toronto so we had to depend on one another for friendship and companionship. This is when we started playing games like backgammon, cribbage, scrabble, and dominoes to pass the time on the weekends.

Denis was excited to start his schooling, as was I for him, and we were excited to set up home in our own apartment. We were incredibly naïve. Little did we know, we had a lot to learn yet.

We hadn't been in Toronto long before I found a job. In fact, when we were in Toronto in August to find this very apartment, I had noticed a job opening for a cook at a restaurant and I told my mother I'd probably get a job there. I was so naïve to think a job would still be there two months following.

After unpacking and settling in, I jumped on a bus and made my way to the restaurant. I spoke with the kitchen manager and filled out an application. She spoke to me at great length about what types of equipment I had worked with as well as my experience. She was quite impressed with what I knew. I guess all those years working in the restaurant for my parents were about to pay off. I got the job, just like that!

When I got home from that interview, I called Mom to tell her I got the job and that my hours would be Monday to Friday, 9 to 5. She didn't believe me and thought I was lying to make her feel better. What a hoot! "No Mom, it's true. I got the job and I start tomorrow," I said.

My mother had been working seven days a week, night and day, in the restaurant for years so she had a hard time believing that I could get a day shift job.

Our apartment turned out to be in a very bad neighborhood, Sirens were part of the normal street noise and for a small-town girl, that took some getting used to. It was not safe to be out on my own at night in this area, or at least that's how I felt at the time. Our car got broken into so often that eventually we left it unlocked. Once our little one's car seat was stolen. We had very little money so from then on, we carried the car seat up to our apartment as we couldn't afford to keep replacing it. Another time, I got home from work and found our home had been ransacked! I was terrified as Denis was not home. He was on a school break and decided to make a quick visit back home to see family and friends. He returned immediately to us once he found out. He has always been our protector, that man.

I worked at the restaurant until 1983. By then, the team had changed quite a bit. The establishment had been bought out and it just wasn't the same anymore. I went to work at my daughter's daycare as a teacher's assistant. We had terrific fun there and when they found out I could cook for a group, they took full advantage of it. I played cook occasionally when the regular one would call in sick. I'm rather certain that she did it on purpose once she knew I was capable. I didn't mind one bit as I love to feed people, especially children. I learned a lot working there and made some very nice friends.

To pass the time while living in Toronto, we'd either hop on the bus, head downtown, ride the subway and people watch, or we'd go to one of the large parks for a walk. For city folks, this would have been boring, but for us, it was enlightening, to say the least. Oh, we'd do a bit of shopping at the Eaton Centre or sometimes we'd head to Kensington or the St. Lawrence Markets and pick up a few things but really we had very little money and we stretched it out as well as we could. I don't think we ever went hungry, but we certainly didn't have many extras.

I remember this one time when we had the police in our apartment writing up a report as our car had been broken into again. I offered the policeman a coffee, but we had no sugar. We had milk but it was only for our little one, and he must have seen me debating mentally whether I should offer him milk or not because he told me he'd take his coffee black. I thought, well, she'll get her milk tonight after all.

The one thing that was constant while living in Toronto was the loneliness I felt being away from my family. Being separated from my siblings and parents was very difficult for me and I missed them terribly. They came to visit occasionally but when they left, I would cry for hours. On our return from an extended Christmas vacation in

1984, as I cried all the way home in the car, we decided it was time to move back. We started to plan the move and got the ball rolling.

You know, today I look back at the young couple that we were and I am proud of them! Those were some very hard days that we had to get through. And we did get through them, together. Maybe what saved us was our evening walks to the park with our daughter. This is where we started what we now call our therapy walks. Every night we take a walk together, just like back then, and discuss any topics or issues that come up during the day. There were no TV's or other distractions, just us. We still do this today. Perhaps we have fewer issues but there are always topics to pick from.

It was during one of these walks that we decided since Denis had a decent job in Toronto, we decided I'd move back to Stoney Point with our little one because I landed a job right away at a factory in Tilbury, Ontario. I was to start right away, so Denis stayed in Toronto to hand in our two months' notice at the apartment and to keep working. Once the two months were up, he moved back to Stoney Point with us and found a job rather quickly at a communications company. It was a great fit for them and him, and he stayed at that job until 1996. He loved working for those people.

Being back in Stoney Point after five years away was a bit of an adjustment but we were so glad to be near friends and family again. For once, we didn't have to plan months in advance to be at certain places, events, etc. It was nice to see Mom whenever I wanted to as well.

Life in Toronto was fine, but we had no family there. In those times, a long-distance phone call home cost us dearly and we didn't dare do it often. We had no computers then either, so there was no Skyping, no e-mails, or Facebook to keep in touch with people. I think I spent my first month home just talking on the phone without any long distance charges!

In the meantime, Denis was finishing up work in Toronto, where he stayed for an extra two months to give final notice to the landlords and to put away a bit of cash.

When Denis landed himself a job with that communications company, we rented a place of our own in Stoney Point. It was a small two-bedroom house, but it was clean, had a huge yard to play in, and was close to family. That's all that mattered to us. It was wonderful to be close to our siblings, parents, and all our friends again. Our little one got to spend more time with her cousins and even was in the same kindergarten class with one of her cousins. That was a bonus for her and she was thrilled.

All was well with the world for us, but maybe we needed to add to the family. It wasn't long after moving back to Stoney Point where we had the itch to add to our family. We got planning and a short time later, we found out we were expecting our second child.

Come October, another girl was welcomed to the world by her very excited parents (Denis and myself) and her big sister. Our new baby weighed in at a whopping 7 pounds, 7 ounces and measured 20 inches long. She weighed all of 1 ounce more than her big sister was at birth and our older daughter was not impressed by this as she figured she should be bigger since she was older.

Our newest addition had many cousins to play with and kept her busy. She was a happy baby and loved the attention lavished on her by her big sister. She would throw her toys around and her big sister would gladly chase them. It was a game neither of them got tired of. She was a very busy toddler often getting into things when we least expected it. Once, when I was making crepes in the kitchen, she somehow got into the drawer in the bathroom. You know the one where you keep all the feminine products right next to the toilet? Anyhow, after about five minutes of not hearing her tear around the house, I called out to the big sister, "Where's the little one?" I first shut off my pan then we started the search. Well, in that short time she had managed to use up a whole box of Stayfree's and had them stuck all over herself, on all of the cabinets, the tub, and even the toilet! When I finally found her in the bathroom hard at work, she looked up at me and said, "Look, Mommy...Stickers!" Now tell me, people, how could you get angry with that innocence?

This little girl has continued to amuse us her entire life. She has a funny way of interpreting happenings, people, and events. She will always let you know what's on her mind and is likely the most generous young woman alive. I continue to be awed by her devotion to God as this is not a popular thing to do in this day and age. Today she is married to a wonderful man and the mother of two beautiful baby girls who bring us so much joy.

Chapter Twelve

THE TRUTH ALWAYS COMES OUT - 1991

Dear Diary,

Phew ... wow, I can't believe Mom finally asked me about Dad. I always said I wouldn't lie if she asked me. Why do I feel as though things are about to get real? Eleven years ago, we, my siblings and I had a meeting to discuss this very thing ... and now it's happening. This much I know for sure, Mom will have her kids back her up 100% and Dad is crazy if he hasn't figured that out. Why did it take Mom so long to see the real Dad? My only answer to that Dear Diary is that she just wasn't ready yet. Her childhood had a real strong hold on her! Also, she has a far higher tolerance level than I do! Moreover she's been a tad distracted with running a crazy busy restaurant and raising eight kids practically single handedly!

It was a nice warm, fall evening and I had just finished making my pickles. The mess was all cleaned up when I heard the doorbell. Looking through the drapes, I noticed Mom's new car, a 1992 Ford. I wondered why she had used the front door and rang the bell rather than use the back door and just walk in as usual. When I opened the door, she motioned to the glider on the front porch and asked if I had a few minutes to talk. So, we sat. I brought out the tea and we talked and talked.

She asked me right off if I ever thought my father had been having an affair. I took a deep breath and answered her honestly. I told her that, yes, I did believe he was having an affair with my Aunt Susie, her sister. She didn't seem surprised, just deeply sad. She went on to tell me that she's been talking with the children and getting their versions of the story as she had been suspecting his affair for a long time. She had always feared she was being manipulated by Dad. Whenever she'd confront Dad about Aunt Susie, he'd say, "How can you think such a thing of your own sister?" His other favorite was, "You have a perverted mind!" She'd feel bad for thinking it and would leave the subject alone. I often wonder how Dad led the double life. Did he ever feel bad? Did he ever realize the pain he caused us all? These are questions that I never got any answers to, but as a parent, I have to believe that he had some realization of it all...at some point. He had to know.

Mom suspected things when Dad would come home late at night and she'd ask why he was so late. He, of course, would say the restaurant was busy but she was no dummy. She'd drive by after closing time, not seeing a single soul or car. He'd still deny it and she'd still believe it, quite simply because it was easier to believe it.

As it turned out, my mom caught on to the fact that my father and Aunt Susie had a disagreement that neither of them could share with Mom and she found out the reason. They'd had a big fight about my aunt's suspicion that he was having an affair with the much younger waitress. Both Mom and Aunt Susie were right on point. Yes, my sixty-year-old Dad was having an affair with a twenty-seven-year-old waitress he employed. She had a husband and two children. Did it bother my father that he was breaking up a family? My father was a very self-involved man, narcissistic some might say, and I'd bet my last dime that he didn't think of these things one bit. He would have made all kinds of excuses and not given it a second thought. He didn't care that he was breaking up two families, his and hers!

This was to be the start of a very intriguing chapter in all of our lives.

Things certainly got interesting in town and in our homes. I am a walker and once the news hit the streets, my walks became a free-for-all by certain people wanting the scoop. People that I hardly knew would be asking me very personal and private questions about my parents.

My sister who was in college at the time actually heard my parents' divorce being discussed while in line at the cafeteria!

This was giving me a new perspective on talking about other people's problems. From then on, I tried keeping any news or gossip that I heard to myself. It's hurtful. I'm sure that none of these people meant to offend, but if I were to run over your foot by accident, it would still hurt, right?

Dad was having a hard time getting support from his kids, as we all recognized the damage he had done to Mom's psyche. Over the years he planted doubt in her mind and had her go against her instincts. It was a real lesson for us all – never grapple against your gut. Your gut is never wrong.

My sister and I wanted to show our support for Mom. It was Halloween night, it was late, wet, cold, and damp. We decided to stake out Dad's place with the help of my sweetie and my brother-in-law. We were dressed in black head-to-toe like we were some kind of spies. We were far from it but we needn't worry. Dad wouldn't think we're capable of this so we could've saved ourselves the trouble. The guys had their thermos' filled with coffee and were staking out the parking lot, waiting for Dad to leave. We all had two-way radios and would call on each other when we noticed any movement on Dad's part. We gave my father the code name "Pinocchio." It was fitting as he liked to tell lies and had a bit of a schnozzle.

My sister and I moved our positions to a field behind Dad's girlfriend's apartment. We were radioed that "Pinocchio" had left his nest and was headed our way. He went into her apartment and he stayed there until 4 a.m. I was starting to get a scratchy throat. Would I make it through the night? I was coughing and making noise, so my sister sent me home where her son was watching our girls.

Our suspicions were confirmed, and it didn't make me feel one bit better. Dad was indeed, once again, having an affair with another woman. Life just got crazier from then on. We wouldn't learn Mom's true feelings about this till a bit down the road. She was still keeping a brave face.

I really wanted this relationship to be a figment of Mom's imagination. I wanted Dad to prove us wrong, but of course, he did not. I would've had much more respect for my father had he left my mother, then started a relationship with whomever he wanted but he didn't...once again.

Chapter Thirteen

WHAT A YEAR – 1992

Dear Diary,

Spring was a tough one for Mom and Dad. First he broke up with Aunt Susie after 25 years of having an affair with her. Then the day after Mother's Day, one of the busiest days of the year at the restaurant, he fired Aunt Susie. Mom was very happy about this but also sad because for all these years, she had tried to convince him to let Aunt Susie go and he wouldn't. Yet a young waitress easily talked him into it. Mom suspected there was something going on, but Dad denied it, of course. Meme D, Mom's mother spoke with Mom regarding the affair and her response was that Aunt Susie was just a girl when it started and didn't know what she was doing. Aunt Susie by now was far beyond being a girl; she was a grown woman. She may have been a young girl when it all started but not anymore. I still wish she had been braver and just left. Turns out, she wished that too. She has huge regrets about not marrying her love, about not staying out when she moved out by believing that Dad loved her and needed her but we all know that Dad didn't truly love her, Dad fills his cup according to his needs.

One summer night after a long and hot shift in the kitchen, Mom went to say good night to Dad, as she often did. She walked into the office to find Dad leaning against the wall and the young waitress was snuggled up against him. Mom was furious and told Dad she was leaving him, but he talked her out of it. In fact, he told her she owed that young waitress an apology for insulting her in that way! So, in tears, Mom apologized to her and asked her to please not leave the restaurant because Dad was worried she'd quit. When Mom revealed this nugget of info, I reminded her that nobody, and I mean nobody, could force her to speak. Why on earth should SHE apologize to that young waitress? That is how manipulative my father was. He would make you feel things you had no business feeling. Why would Mom feel shame for catching them snuggling in the office? That young waitress had no business snuggling another woman's husband and she gets an apology from Mom. Can you say ***wrong?!***

In late September of that same year, Dad came to Mom's bed and asked if he could make love to her. It was the first time in nine years that he had come to her. She thought her patience had paid off and she was elated to share her bed with him.

The next day he asked her if she'd go on a holiday with him. It would be the first time in twenty-seven years that they'd take a trip on their own without children, sisters, or anybody else. They planned a trip to Gatlinburg right after their 39th anniversary. That night, Mom went to the bingo and won $1,000. She was on a lucky streak. She gave Dad half the winnings to spend on the holiday as she was just so excited to be getting away with him at last. She was on cloud nine.

On the day of their anniversary, October 17th, some of my siblings stopped by the restaurant to wish them well on the trip and to bid them a happy anniversary. Dad assured the children that he was sorry for what he had done with Aunt Susie, tears running down his cheeks, saying he'd never do anything like that again.

The day they left for Gatlinburg, Mom was very excited but Dad was noticeably not so much. They made many stops along the way and each time they did, Dad would use his cell phone to call his new favorite waitress. When Mom would get back to the car, she'd ask who he was talking to and he'd say just one of the employees at the restaurant. After catching Dad on the phone with her several times, she asked him if he had anything to tell her. "Not right now I don't," was his reply. She let that comment go by without a retort. Perhaps "please explain, dear" would've been a good place to start with him.

The next day after they did a bit of shopping and touring, Dad sat Mom down and told her that he hadn't loved her in over twenty years. She was astounded and asked him why he took her on a holiday to tell her this. He said that this favorite waitress of his had told him that he should take her on one last trip and had also advised him to go to Mom's room in September and make love to her to determine whether he still loved her or not. Mom was very ticked off!

When Dad fell asleep, she went into his wallet and took back her $500 winnings from the bingo. She figured he didn't deserve it after all. This cracks me up because if this was my husband, I'm not sure I'd go so easy on him. I think I would have grabbed the keys, left him stranded, and let his little girlfriend get him home.

Mom wanted to discuss their marriage and how things would change, but Dad laughed and said there was nothing left to discuss. He genuinely thought that she'd simply put up with him carrying on and living as if nothing happened.

Unfortunately, Dad's planning was not so well-thought-out as they had a 12-hour ride home following that lovely chat from the night before. He told her he wanted to move out but not until after Christmas because he didn't want to ruin the children's holidays. He wanted to wait three months and perhaps he'd love her again by then. She replied that he hadn't loved her in twenty years, what could possibly change in three months? She said that he would have to leave as soon as they got home. Mom was finally getting a backbone and it was feeling good. She was just getting started.

As soon as they got home, Dad went straight to her place, the little waitress's place and then moved to the apartment above the restaurant. That used to be such a beautiful apartment but not so much anymore since Mom and Dad had moved into the lake house. The apartment had fallen into disrepair and had been used mainly for storage for the restaurant! Life was about to change for all of us from then on.

A few days later, Mom bumped into a friend at church. They stood on the steps and chatted. He asked how her trip to Gatlinburg was and she filled him in on Dad's revelation that he didn't love her anymore. Mom's friend seemed stunned. He walked back to the restaurant with Mom, and they sat and had a coffee and a dish of rice pudding. Dad sat down and joined them.

This good friend asked Dad what his main issue was regarding their marriage. Dad's brilliant response was that Mom was always paying attention to the children and not him. Mom's friend sat in shock and finally asked Dad, "If not for her, who would pay attention to the children?"

That was a good point that Dad had never considered. He was always so busy looking after his needs that our needs or Mom's were never much of a thought to him. He honestly believed that saying his wife paid attention to his children instead of him was a sound reply and a respectable reason for having an affair with his sister-in-law for twenty-five years, then starting up a new affair with another young woman, all the while married to the mother of his eight kids. Eight kids that he helped conceive by the way.

Chapter Fourteen

STAY OFF THE SIDEWALKS!

Dear Diary,

Well, Diary, Mom has gone off the rails! Oh my! I feel as if she's had 60 years of emotional baggage piling up and she is about to blow like a volcano! I am worried about her; she's behaving in an erratic fashion. My older siblings took Mom on a trip to London to see her family Dr., they toured the psychiatric hospital in St. Thomas to scare her straight, which seems to have worked ... or is she just faking it for them? My brother has been sleeping at her place to keep an eye on her. I think this is helping her as she's less lonely. Let's hope between that and her appointments with her therapist that she'll come around to her normal self again. I hope I never see the inside of a jail again!

Mom was working in her hot kitchen, prepping/breading her fish for the evening shift. It was a Tuesday and that meant the famous Yellow Perch or Lake Erie Pickerel dinners would be on special tonight, so plenty of fish would be needed. This was a house specialty at the Stoney Point Tavern where regulars patronized on their favorite day of the week based on the daily special. One day it was the famous Broasted chicken, another day fish, then their smoked baby back ribs brought in many people on Wednesdays plus the homemade soup and salad bar that came with all meals were a real draw for our extremely busy restaurant.

Dad came into the kitchen, which was a rare occasion unless he came in to complain about something. He proceeded to throw a steak on the charcoal broiler. My father rarely ate red meat and this surprised my mother as he was not exactly the generous type so she knew he wouldn't be giving it away. She asked him who the steak was for. He said it was for his favorite young waitress. She hasn't had anything to eat all day and it was past three o'clock in the afternoon. Mom replied, "Since when do we give steaks to the staff? Fix her a burger or give her soup and salad like the rest of the staff gets!" Dad never liked being told what to do and he told her that should mind her own business, to which she replied, "This ***is*** my business!" It made her very angry because he had always griped about her giving their own kids free lunches...and here he was cooking a T-bone steak for this very young and attractive woman. Mom knew there was something suspicious going on. This time she was listening to her gut.

Shortly after the steak was served, Dad was sitting with this young waitress when she said, "Oh, I have to go meet the kids at the bus. The sitter won't get there for another fifteen minutes or so." Dad said, "No, you finish your steak. I'll meet them at the bus." When Mom noticed Dad had left, she asked where he'd gone. When Mom realized he'd gone to meet the waitress's kids at the bus, it angered her tremendously that Dad was doing this.

Why would this anger Mom, you may ask? Well, only recently Mom had received a call from one of her kids who was stuck in Windsor and asked Mom to pick up their daughter at school. Dad responded, "Are we running a daycare now, too?" It really ticked Mom off that he ran out to pick up a staff member's kids while his little four-year-old granddaughter was going to be stranded at school and he didn't want my mother to pick her up! She tore out of the restaurant and jumped into her car and raced out of the parking lot.

She headed down Main Street, which is not a long trip if you knew the size of this village. She spotted Dad walking on the sidewalk. As an overpowering anger overcame her, she jumped her car over the curb and then came flying down the sidewalk, heading straight for Dad. My father saw her coming towards him and started running. Mom stopped within inches of running him over or throwing him into the plate-glass window of the supermarket. My father yelled at her and told her to get back to the restaurant immediately. So like a good wife, she meandered back to the restaurant. Old habits die hard; she obeyed him and headed back to the restaurant.

Mom was waiting for Dad in the office. When he came marching in, madder than a soaked cat, he proceeded to yell at her. She wasn't going to take it! She hauled off and socked him right across the side of his face. The young waitress heard the ruckus and came running to Dad's rescue, but Mom slammed the door in her face and told her to mind her own business. She was afraid of Mom and, not being completely stupid, left them to settle things on their own. Dad was left with a huge goose egg on the side of his face and his pride somewhat bruised. He was angry and he came back at Mom. He shook her and she banged her head against the wall a couple of times. They both got their licks in and then continued right back to work like nothing at all had happened.

Astonishingly, Mom returned to the kitchen and finished her shift. Nothing more was said or done about the incident for months to come. Not even her children had heard of this incident...yet.

A couple of months later, someone had scratched the waitress' car. It was a long huge scratch all along the side of the car and that same person had put a few bags of garbage in her car as well. She and Dad called the police and when the two young policewomen showed up, Dad poured his heart out about the sidewalk experience. He gave them all the details, omitting the part about him having an affair with a woman thirty-three years his junior. They took that information back to their captain, and after having heard everything, the captain issued a warrant to have Mom picked up for attempted vehicular manslaughter.

I was preparing a pot of beef stew when Mom called to say she wouldn't be making it for dinner. I could tell by her voice that she was still very upset and having a bad day. I said, "Nonsense, you get your butt down here and I'll put the kettle on." She said I'd have to invite along the police officers that were taking her away. You could have knocked me over with a feather!

Her explanation was that she'd had car trouble and her car had jumped the curb, curiously at the very same moment when Dad had been walking on that very sidewalk. Oh, My M.O.M!

I asked her where the police were taking her and she said, "The Essex detachment. Call your sister." She would know what to do. I called my sister, gave her the details, and from there we found out Mom would be fingerprinted, her mug shot would be taken, and she was to be transferred to the Windsor police station waiting for her case to be heard before a judge. Mug shot of my sweet Mom? How is this even a part of a sentence? I was struggling to accept all this information as it didn't fit in my head. Mom would never harm anyone. This is nuts! I was feeling stressed, angry with Dad, hurt for Mom – I was just in a puddle of emotions.

We made plans to drive to Windsor to pick her up. Well, in reality, ***to bail her out!*** Mom had been acting a bit odd lately and this just didn't make sense. We still didn't know the story. We haven't heard the real story yet from Mom. There had to be some sort of explanation.

We all decided to meet Mom at the Windsor jail. I drove with my sister but before she picked me up, I made a quick call to the restaurant to speak with Dad but was told he was at the garage. His nephew owned the local garage and often Dad would go there to chinwag with him.

I phoned the Garage and my cousin passed the phone over to Dad. I let him have it with both barrels. I was so angry that he would call the police on Mom after all the crap he put her through. He had some kind of nerve. I let him know that he wasn't going to sweet talk me into believing his crap a second longer. I told him how I heard him coming into my room when I was just three years old and what kind of father would ever do that to a child or his young sister-in-law, by the way? He shouted that he'd had enough. "Really, have you Dad?" I said. "I was only getting started!" I was fuming. All these years my mother was the good wife, put up with all his shenanigans, worked tirelessly to make that restaurant not only busy but amazingly successful, and he gets her put in jail? The balls on this guy! I mean, you have to admit, he had game. His only flaw in his thinking was that now that he had her arrested, the whole story was about to hit the local gossips. Word was spreading like the H1N1 virus!

My sister picked me up in her red car shortly after all the phone calls and off we went to Windsor, a 45-minute drive for us. The conversation on the way to the jail was somber, to say the least. We were both concerned as neither of us had any experience being locked up. We just didn't know what to expect. I kept saying there's got to be a mistake; something is not right about this. I asked my sister if she'd seen signs that Mom was perhaps losing her grip on reality. My very intuitive sister uttered that a person can only take so much stress and perhaps Mom had maxed out her limit.

My two other sisters, coming directly from work, met us at the Windsor jail. We arrived at the station and I was surprised by the normalcy of the reception area. It almost seemed like a doctor's office. I soon came to the realization of where I was when I heard Mom in her cell giving the policemen a hard time and likely a good laugh. Here was this sixty-year-old woman who looked about as dangerous as a soft little kitten yelling at them that she had to pee! She finally pulled her pants down and told them all to enjoy the show. She was shouting, "You want to see my big fat ass, then have a look, boys!" She used the urinal or what she thought was a urinal. My sisters' concern was to make sure the officers were aware that Mom was diabetic and that she would need apple juice.

I was trying to come to grips with all this. I kept thinking who is that woman and what have they done with Mom? While sitting in the middle of the lobby of the police station, I was feeling an out of body experience. I stood up and announced to everyone in the lobby, "I feel the need to tell you all that my mother is a good woman. She has led a good life, but she is having trouble right now!" Phew, that felt good. The world needed to know that.

My sisters asked me if I'd lost my mind, to which I answered, "Maybe I have!" One sister kept telling me to shut up, another was trying to sit me down, and the third was on the floor laughing, as this was often her nervous reaction to situations.

The scene was something out of a *Twilight Zone* episode for me. It was all too surreal as though I was outside my body watching from somewhere else and not able to stop this runaway train called Mom. She was on a path to destruction and I could not find the brakes! It was a nightmare that I could not wake from. I certainly didn't expect ***that day***; we'd have to bail our sweet mother from jail. And did I turn off the stew? The ride home was a quiet one for us all. Mom tried to explain why she was so angry and once she told us about Dad going to the bus stop for that waitress's kids, I got it. I assured her we'd be there to help her sort all this out and her kids would always support her 100%.

In the weeks following, the only comfort that I could offer Mom was tea. I vowed that I would have Mom over often for tea and I did just that. She wasn't able to come every day, but she came whenever possible. When she did show up, we would have the best chats over that pot of tea. That was how I felt I could help, just by listening to her and letting her vent. She had so much anger pent up from all those years of being denied her feelings. On one of our tea dates, she would tell me that long ago she believed that Dad was having an affair with Aunt Susie and Dad would shame her for even asking him. "How can you think that of me or your sister? Shame on you!" he'd say.

My father was a master manipulator and at last, he had no more hold on her. She was letting it all out. Boy oh boy, was she letting it all out!

In the end, after a very interesting trial, her defense attorney extraordinaire defended Mom with the battered person syndrome.

Dad may not have physically abused Mom, but he verbally abused her all of their married life. All their children were willing to testify if need be. He was forever calling her names; his favorite term was "stupid." He called her that repeatedly. The trial ended and Mom was given a year of probation with community service.

She chose to work at the soup kitchen downtown and she served the best soup those homeless people ever had! She did her time as she did everything, with passion and ardor.

Mom would not be victimized again. In fact, it became her motto: "I will not be victimized again!" Put that on a t-shirt, she'd say!

This chapter in Mom's life was a huge learning lesson to all that loved her. First, there was the lesson that a child mistreated will carry that burden for life, and because of that, I believe we are all better parents.

The next lesson was to believe in yourself. Nobody knows you like you! If you strongly sense something, inquire about it. If you still don't feel satisfied, inquire till you do. Do not be manipulated into doing things that you have no business doing.

Chapter Fifteen

MOM MEETS FRED – 1994

Dear Diary,

My mother is dating! Can my world get any weirder? I finally got to meet Fred. He seems like a very nice man. He sure seems to like Mom, who wouldn't? It seems that Mom likes him, so I think they'll be fine. I'm glad things are coming together for her. She seems to be moving on with life. I see many more smiles than I've seen in a while; this is all good, right? Remind me to tell him not to tick her off!

In the spring of 1994 when Mom was feeling stronger, she started dating. There was one fellow who shall remain nameless, and he definitely was memorable to Mom. They had been dating here and there, getting along well. One day when he was at her place for dinner, the phone rang. It was one of her children. She answered the phone and engaged in a conversation. When she got off the phone, he asked her, "Who comes first, me or your children?" She got up, took his plate, threw it in the sink, and told him to get out! I guess that answered that question. Nobody questioned Mom's love for her children...***ever!*** She told him, "Those kids were here a hell of a lot longer than you have been. Here's your hat. ***Get out!***" Mom was empowered, and it was thrilling!

In August of 1994, she met Fred. They found each other in the Pennysaver, a local newspaper with dating ads. Mom answered his ad the old-fashioned way, via snail mail. They had met only a week prior to her going on vacation with my sister and her family, and she would be gone for two weeks. During that trip, they toured Canada's West, camping and making their way around Alberta. They all had a blast together.

The day before Mom returned from that trip, Fred convinced my brother to let him in her house. He bought vases of roses that he placed all over her house. He was very excited for her to get home. Following her return home, they dated more frequently. They went on long rides and shared mutual stories about their exes, their children, their work, etc. They hit it off fantastically! He was becoming a great companion to have around. I remember one day she called me and asked me for my meatloaf recipe. I thought it funny as I usually called her for recipes, but she said she loved my meatloaf. So, I shared my recipe and apparently, Fred loved it as well.

Fred moved into Mom's home just before Christmas of 1994 and they began a life together. They would go to all the nearby farmers' markets and get the best local produce. They canned tomatoes, pickles, peaches, beets, and any other vegetables or fruits that made it to their kitchen. They were a team of sorts. They spent their evenings playing cards and capping the night off with the news as though they'd been married for years.

It didn't take Mom long to figure out she needed some time to herself. She spent so many of her hours caring for others that this would be a day that she did as she pleased, when she pleased. She didn't do it often but when she did, she'd usually be gone for the day. It was on one of these days that she had an experience that would go down in history as one of the funniest stories she ever told, and oh how she loved telling it. I loved Mom's stories.

She said to me, "It was a beautiful spring day and after weeks of caring and doing for others, I decided to take a "Bev" day. I started out with a bit of shopping just browsing without anybody rushing me and looking at what I wanted at a pace I liked. I wasn't shopping for anything that I needed." She was simply just passing time.

Then she said, "I went and had a pizza buffet for lunch." She liked this on her Bev day as there'd be little interaction with servers because sometimes a girl just needs to be alone. She was constantly surrounded by family, friends, and also at the time, Fred.

My mother was a closet celiac. Her mother was celiac, her daughter is, her granddaughter is, and her great-granddaughters are! Did she think the gene skipped her generation? She was never diagnosed with it but then again, she never presented it to her doctors. Every time she'd have certain foods, especially containing gluten, she'd have reactions.

That day, she had her fill of gluten, I mean pizza, pasta, salad, and even a bit of dessert. She was a happy camper and was ready to play bingo. She was feeling lucky! She got in the car and started heading towards the Bingo hall.

As it turned out, she said "That wasn't luck I was feeling! Suddenly, my tummy was in agony. The gas and the tightening of my belly was telling me to get to a toilet and fast!" She pulled into the closest place to her location, which was a department store. She knew the store well and they had a washroom on the main level. She rushed for it, hoping there'd be nobody in it as it was a single-use washroom.

She said, "Luckily there was nobody in it! I got my pants pulled down just in time to splatter the walls, toilet, floor, and just about anything in splashing distance! It was horrible!" She said she sat on that toilet until her belly felt somewhat better. That's when she heard a woman in the hall loudly explaining to a small child that surely the woman in the washroom must be almost done! Oh no! Not a child.

She tried to clean up the best she could, wiping down the walls, the toilet seat, and the floor with paper towels. There was some type of cleaning spray in the bathroom, so she sprayed it with hopes that it would mask the smell but, alas, nothing could mask that smell! She did the best she could and walked out with her eyes averted so as not to see their faces when they walked in.

She decided to go to bingo anyway. After all, she had cleaned herself up and tossed her undies, so she thought, "Why not?" What could possibly be worse than that? She headed for the Bingo hall.

Once she got organized, got her cards laid out, her dabbers all tested and ready to go, she relaxed and thought, "There, I'm all set to win now!" As she was finally relaxing, she could detect the faint smell of poop and wondered if it was on one of her shoes. No, it wasn't her shoes. Um...maybe a pant leg? No, it wasn't there. She decided to let it go.

She continued to tell me this story. "After a while of playing and dabbing, it was starting to annoy me. Where was that smell coming from? I dabbed my card and that's when I saw it! I had shit all down my sleeve, I mean right to the elbow! I had been playing with an arm covered in shit! No bloody wonder I was sitting alone!"

I was laughing so hard I nearly had an accident myself! I had to ask, "Mom what did you do next?" She said, "I was horrified and ran out of there like a cat on fire! I can never go back to that Bingo hall!"

My mother was an awesome storyteller and she told everyone this story so I am not breaking any kind of family secrets by sharing this. She would love to watch people when she told this story. Oh, how she had a great laugh.

Mom would go on to have many more of these stories and she'd happily share them over a bowl of soup, over the telephone, or standing in line at the grocery store. She absolutely thought they were funny.

Although it's funny to hear these stories, I suggest that if this happens often to you, then perhaps it's time to get that looked after. It's not good for one's body to go through this on a regular basis. There is definitely something going on with you that needs looking after. Please, I beg you, look after yourself. People love you and need you.

Mom's "Bev" days would be limited for a time as shortly thereafter, Fred had his first heart attack. He gave the whole family quite a scare but seemed to get things under control. Then again in 1996, he had his second, the big one. The ambulance took him away and he had a third one on the way to the hospital. Fred ended up being transferred to the Detroit hospital as they were better equipped for the issues he was experiencing. He suffered yet another heart attack on his way over there. Somehow, they stabilized him and got him on the right medications and back on track.

This was a turning point for Fred. He could have jumped tracks, got into better shape, learned better eating habits, or just get some exercise but he'd have none of it, no matter how much mom nagged him. Instead, he chose to sit in his recliner and not do much of anything except watch TV and eat, all day long. He even stopped his woodworking. Up until this point, he would spend hours in the garage creating all kinds of beautiful pieces. He made clocks, shelves, captain benches, and just about anything that was asked of him. He had a definite gift for this. He did very little of his woodworking afterward, a craft that not only he was good at, but he loved doing. He seemed to have lost hope in life. However, I'm pleased to report that he taught my brother, who is now carrying on the tradition of woodworking. He's created a few beauties himself lately!

Fred, though, was a constant companion to Mom and they got along well. I don't think it was a case of mad love. They were compatible and it worked for them. On November 2, 2002, they finally tied the knot. They had many grown grandkids by then and Mom said she wanted to set an example for everyone and to make it legal. They had a simple wedding with their entire family in attendance and had a lovely reception.

After their wedding, life didn't change much. They stuck to their same old routines and nothing could convince Fred to go out for a walk. This would later prove to be detrimental to Mom as she was bypassing on her walks too. She was putting her health on the line and the more we tried talking to her about taking walks, the more closed she got about it. She was not taking care of herself and it was beginning to show. Her health seemed to be on a slow decline but she was in denial.

Fred would go on to exist another six years. I say exist because that's what it is when you're not living. Living is being out and about and doing things with friends and family, taking part in hobbies, crafts, sports, or whatever it is that tickles your fancy. Mom was afraid if she left Fred home, he'd die on her. And yet each day, it took a little more of Mom's health. She would bring food to him rather than have him get up and move a bit at least. He was losing feeling in his feet, then his legs.

He started falling because he had no feeling in his legs now. He was a big man, at least 300 pounds, and my mother would help him up. Mom ended up with six hernias and need an operation. The specialist told her after the surgery, "You are not to help that man get up ever again. Do you understand?" To my knowledge, she never did. So from then on when Fred fell, she'd call the local fire department. They'd come over and it took two or three large firefighters to get him upright. Here she had been doing this on her own!

The lesson here people is to take care of your health while you have it! Don't wait till you start having heart attacks. Eat well, get active, and live life to its fullest. Do you really want to burden anyone with your care if you can prevent it? There are times in life where we get illnesses and we need help. That is a different thing altogether. Most of Fred's problems stemmed from a life of indulgences and absolutely no activity.

There are so many activities we can choose from in today's society! Do you like to swim? Most towns and cities have pools, tennis courts, hockey arenas, and places to walk (which is cheap). Zumba is fun and pickleball is very popular now. Just pick something and give it a whirl. If you don't like it, try something else. But don't stop! The worst thing we can do is just sit in front of the TV all day and night. Turn that thing off and go for a stroll. Maybe walk your neighbor's dog, you know the one who's confined to the house while its owners are at work. Like the sports ad says: just do it!

Chapter Sixteen

THE MOVE TO LONDON – 1996

Dear Diary,

Well, here we go, Diary! Everything is packed, thanks to Denis and our little girl. While we were in London Monday to Friday, they were here packing up! The cargo bin is full, and in the morning the truck will arrive to deliver it to our new address! Woot woot! The younger daughter is pumped about the pool; the older daughter is pumped to going back to her new friends in London. I feel like our world is shifting, in a good way. It's been a rough few years with all that went on with Mom and Dad; now it's time to take time for us. Wish me luck, Diary...

After a year of working in the food service sales as a distributor Rep in Windsor, my job was eliminated. I immediately began job searching and found that another Distributor was looking for a rep for the London area. I faxed over a resume and immediately got a call. Could I come in for an interview? They were a company located in Kitchener and serviced the South West area of Ontario. With all that had been going on with Mom and Dad, we needed a change at home. Denis and I discussed it and we decided that I'd take the job if they offered it to me.

I arrived all dressed up and ready for the interview, feeling confident and ready to take on the world. After a short meeting, they offered me the job, which I accepted right on the spot. There was no need to mull it over.

Since the position was in London, it meant picking up stakes and leaving friends and family behind to move two hours away, but somehow I felt it was the right choice. At times, the toughest decisions to make are the right ones and in this case, we were right. We put our house on the market and by spring it was sold.

While our house was for sale in Stoney Point, I was living in London with my sister-in-law and her husband. They put up with me for eight whole months. At the time, they only had one daughter, and we bonded on Tuesday nights when they went out to a meeting together. My niece and I would eat chips and watch TV. I'd get her in bed just before the parents got home. It was a special time for us.

We believed we had found our new home, so we had our older daughter come stay with me in London to start her second semester at school. It turned out we didn't get that house after all, but she did complete a semester in the new school before summer which helped her to make friends earlier than expected. Things always happen for a reason.

Finally, after the 1996 school year ended, we moved to London, Ontario. The move itself was a ton of work, as they normally are. Mom and Fred helped us out as much as they could, and Mom brought a date nut loaf, Meme D's recipe, to nibble on while we worked.

To help with the heavy lifting, our daughter invited a friend from school. He was a huge help and we filled him with as much pizza as he could eat or until we ran out. I don't remember which.

This was an important and emotional move for us as we had a ten-year-old and a sixteen-year-old. This is not always easy to accomplish because, at those ages, they've made friendships that are quite established. Nonetheless, we moved, and the girls quickly made new friends with a bit of encouragement here and there.

In fact, in early July I was putting the garbage to the curb when a young girl around ten years of age walked by with a group of her friends. Forgetting that I was a stranger to her, I asked her how old she was. I think I scared the girl because today she'd likely tell you a different story. Coming from a small town, you know your neighbors, and I forgot for a minute that we were now living in a large city. I told this young girl that we had a ten-year-old daughter, we had just moved here, and our daughter wanted to make some friends. They invited our little girl out to play soccer with them at the park and from then on, they were friends. I can't imagine today talking to a child and saying, "Come to my house and I'll introduce you to my little girl." That poor child must've thought me nuts.

Later that fall, our older daughter who never gave us any trouble went out with her new friends. They were going to the Lambeth Fall fair and would be home by 11 p.m., her curfew time. She was never late, a consummate people pleaser and tonight she was...late. We were sitting on the porch in the dark waiting for her. I was worried and knew instinctively something was wrong. We saw a cab pull up kitty-corner to our house when three teens got out, two of them were boys and one was a very drunk young lady. We could not see them clearly yet other than their shadowy figures in the dark, but I knew it was my girl. When they got to the porch, the boys were holding her up and did not see us because of the bushes in front of the porch. They were telling her to stand up straight and to be cool. When they got to the porch, Denis said, "Hello boys, what have you got there?" I thought they'd pee their pants from the fright of it all!

Her boyfriend told us that they had been drinking and she had decided to drink rye straight without any kind of mix. Now let me tell you a bit about our girl's size. She is 5 3 and weighs about 100 pounds soaking wet. I'm pretty sure after about two of those shots she would have been polluted but she didn't stop at two. She, of course, got quite ill and her boyfriend said he stayed by her side the whole time and had her purse with him as well. A real prince I thought. My husband Denis offered to give the boys a ride home but for some reason, they declined and ran for the hills. Denis had a way of looking very stern when he needed to and those boys were taking no chances at all. Probably the wisest choice they made all night.

Denis carried our girl to bed and our quiet little princess told us she loved us, repeatedly, and that we were the best parents in the world. I think the liquor was talking for her.

Our daughter has never given us a moment of worry since that night. In fact, she was an honor roll student and went on to graduate from university with a bachelor's degree in psychology. She is now married to a wonderful man, and she's a fantastic mother herself with two beautiful children, a boy and a girl. I see her parenting and I am awed at her patience. She is a very good mother and I am so very proud of her. I pray that my parenting was good enough because we were so young when we had her. We certainly gave it our best shot. We read many books about raising children and we discussed parenting often with people whom we admired with child-rearing skills.

Chapter Seventeen

WORKING IT! – 1998 TO 2000

Dear Diary,

I've come up with this ingenious idea to increase my sales, make my customers happy and to get my boss off my back! I swear he's harassing me with his constant phone calls. It's as if he thinks I can force people into buying more; they only need what they need. He has all kinds of tricks to make more profit. I don't know how much more I can take. I really should talk to Denis about this. I feel as if I'm going to blow a gasket here. But I think if I do this blitz, I could increase my sales and finally get him off my rear. You think? I really hope so anyway!

In the fall of 1998, I was recruited by another food distributor, asking me if I'd like to meet for an interview. I was growing tired of this particular distributor taking over a lot of my customers, so I thought if you can't beat them, join them. By the spring of 2000, I had been with this new distributor for almost two years and now had Bayfield as part of my territory. If you've never been to Bayfield, then you should plan something soon. It's a small cottage community on Lake Huron, where every night the most spectacular sunset awaits you! They call it Ontario's West Coast.

My trip would take me to Bayfield on Tuesday mornings, where I'd spend the day in the area and stay the night at a customer's place. She was an eccentric artist who was also a chef for one of my accounts at the time. She had an extra room and rented it out to me on most Tuesdays. Then I would head out on Wednesday mornings and spend another full day in the area seeing all the people I missed the day before. My territory included many restaurants, camps, and hotels that were my customers in this area, so it took me two days to see them all.

In the spring of 2000, I had talks with a food broker rep who was doing some work on my behalf for my customers. We had lunch and I told her that I thought it would be great to get a bunch of reps up here to do this all at once. Then we could stay the night, meet for dinner, and make it a work/play thing. She thought it ingenious, so I got to work.

I invited eight women, all manufacturer reps or brokers who represented products that we sold at our distributor. Once I had heard that they'd all be coming, I booked appointments for everyone over a period of two days. They were each seeing at least five customers per day and would likely be doing good sales since I had presold the customers on the products. Their bosses were thrilled and then I realized maybe I should let my boss in on this plan of mine.

I contacted my sales manager and let him know what I was up to. He thought it sounded very good. In fact, he must have bragged about it to the president because I got an e-mail that week thanking me for my ingenuity. What I hadn't counted on was the boss man coming to town while we were in mid-blitz.

On day number one, all the ladies did very well. When we met for dinner that first night, the table was abuzz with chatter of glory stories. Suddenly, the room went completely quiet. I turned my head to see my boss standing at the end of the table. He was in a muscle shirt with his tattoos on display, and then one of my friends said, "Hey, how many packs of bubble gum did you have to chew to get that tattoo?" The room broke into laughter and I couldn't help but smile while noticing he was not. Women can be spiteful when they want to be.

All of the customers were pleased with me as they hadn't been given this much attention from vendors in a long time. The sales reps were thrilled that their two days of appointments were fully booked for them to facilitate the sale of contracted products for the busy summer ahead. My boss was very pleased. I had a 37% rise in sales for the first week alone! It's all about the numbers in sales and at this point, I was a superstar.

I decided to do it again in the spring of 2001 and that year I added more vendors, both male and female, and we even had T-shirts made. I had the vendors sponsor the T-shirts by buying a space on them. They had prizes for the customers, samples, and loot bags. It was another huge success for me and I was feeling quite confident about my workplace. Silly me.

Unfortunately, all good things come to an end. The moment those planes hit the Twin Towers, my numbers took a dive and it all went to hell in a handbasket from then on. The whole Huron County area depended greatly on our American friends for their economy and the 9/11 events brutally affected their business; which in turn affected mine in an enormous way. I lost my job on November 11, 2001. Exactly two months after 9/11. At the time I was devastated as I had put a lot of pride in my job and based my self-worth on my work. I knew I did a good job and that my customers loved me but that wasn't enough. The events of 9/11 had a huge impact on much of the world and for my sector. In our area, because we bordered the USA, heads had to roll and mine was just one of many.

I didn't realize just how stressed out I was by this job until I wasn't working. I took some time off, taking advantage of the severance pay. I learned to paint, or tried, I cooked massive amounts of food and often, and I exercised to make up for all that cooking. Plus, I still searched high and low for a job.

Then one day I got a call from an industry friend asking me if I had found work yet. He was the manufacturer rep for a company that made muffin and cookie doughs. I told him I had not and right there, he asked me to come and work part-time for him. He offered me a decent wage, a car allowance, and I would be working Tuesday through Thursday. It was an offer I could not refuse.

This turned out to be one of my favorite jobs and he was an amazing boss. He would give me tasks, I'd do them, and we'd carry on. Having a freezer full of cookie dough and muffin batter samples was just a bonus. Apparently, our youngest daughter enjoyed that cookie dough more than I knew. Chocolate Chunk cookies were one of our family's favorites and I was their new hero.

On a very cold but clear March morning (there was no snow for once but it was definitely cold), I was headed to Kitchener, Ontario to do a demonstration on the cookie and muffin line. The back seat of my car was packed with fresh-baked cookies and muffins and the front seat covered in brochures. I had my music going and was settled in for an hour's drive along Highway 401 eastbound listening to my music and mentally planning my demonstration when I noticed all the trucks were moving into the center lane. This is unusual for Highway 401 but I continued along and moved over to the "gunner" lane or the passing lane.

I was moving along at a fast pace when all at once I hit black ice and my car started to skid. The back end of my car collided with a semi-truck which sent my car flying into the guard rail, causing even more consequences. From there I bounced off the guard rail back into the same semi, damaging my right front fender. I was terrified that this would be my last day on Earth. Had I said I love you to my daughter on the way out the door? Did I tell my husband I love him when he left this morning? When was the last time I spoke to my older girl? Did I tell her how proud I was of her? All these things came to mind as I bounced back at the guard rail, now having damaged three corners of my poor car.

This last collision threw me back into danger. The nose of my car was heading straight into the center of the semi! Fearing for my life, I did what any sensible woman would do – I closed my eyes. I heard another crash and braced myself for the worse, fearing this was my last thought on earth.

I know you'll find this hard to believe, and that's okay...I know the truth...I felt a large pair of hands clasp over mine, turn the wheel back, and somehow guided me back to safety on the shoulder of the highway. This large pair of hands could have been imagined or perhaps they were my guardian angel. Either way, I was grateful for the help.

When I opened my eyes, my foot was still hard on the brake pedal, car still in drive and running. I was terrified to look in the mirror for fear that I'd be covered in blood. I finally did, and I could not see any bruises or blood...phew, what a relief!

After locating my cell phone among the scattered cookies, muffins, and brochures, I called 911 and reported the accident. Help was on the way. I had some pain in my chest and they sent an ambulance to look me over.

Having just experienced the closest call of my life, I decided to contact my beloved husband to tell him of my terrifying adventure. When he answered the phone, in a trembling voice I told him of my accident and he asked if I was alright. Before I could answer him, my cell phone died!

Denis was panicked! Having heard of the accident on the radio by traffic scanners, he raced to the scene in his work van and came to me with open arms. I was stoic until this moment, but the tears started the second I saw Denis. How is it that a grown woman can be brave until she spots her husband and then all at once melts into a puddle of tears? He was relieved to see I was unhurt other than a bruise to my chest, thanks to my lifesaving seat belt. Once the medics looked me over and released me, he drove me home to safety and made me a warm cup of relaxing camomile tea.

Upon arrival at home, our youngest daughter was horrified that I had been in an accident and said that she'd had a bad feeling when I left for work that morning. She had worked the night shift and when she came in that morning, she asked me to be careful on my way to Kitchener. We should listen to our instincts more often.

Our older daughter was visibly shaken when she heard the news. "What if you had been taken from us?" she said. "Our future children would have no grandmother. We would have no mother. Mom, you have to be more careful." From that day forward, I took a whole new look at life and at what is important to me. Suddenly, driving all over Ontario to promote cookies and muffins was no longer important. ***Being alive was!***

My car was totaled and written off, while the semi-tractor trailer carrying pigs to their own destinies had barely suffered a scratch. I found it ironic that my last name is Bacon and of all the trucks to hit, I choose one that was carrying pigs.

Miraculously I only had a bruise across my chest without any other lasting effects. To this day, I believe that my life was spared for a reason and wonder daily why exactly that is. I hope to find that out soon enough.

I also thank God that I have lived to see my grandchildren being brought into this world of ours. I cannot imagine my life without them or theirs without me! Who would teach them to bake cookies, teach them French, or make playdough with them? Luckily, I get to do those things and more.

I worked for that company for three years and to this day, I'm still on great terms with my former boss. He was always supportive and respectful, which can't be said for all my bosses until that point in my life.

I was sad to leave them for a full-time position and to this day, I regret making that move. But at the time, I had a daughter starting university and the wage offered was far too tempting.

The lesson here is to not always base a life decision on money alone. I wish I had taken more time to research the job offered to me. Did I really want all the responsibilities? I did finally learn that just because a person offers you a job doesn't mean you have to accept it.

Part Three

TRAGEDY, SADNESS, JOY,
PEACE, ENDINGS

Chapter Eighteen

MY NEPHEW DAVID'S ACCIDENT – 2003

July 11,2003

Dear Diary,

Oh my, oh my, oh my. What do I do? I cannot imagine what my sister is feeling right now. I just can't believe this is happening, how is it even possible? He's 25! I can't believe I won't ever see those blue eyes again; he'll never prank me or anyone else ever again. How is this possible? I am so terribly sad, I can't stop crying, how can I go away and have a weekend with Denis when I am feeling this way? Even if I don't go to Toronto, I'm not going to Stoney Point to see my sister until our daughter is home ... ugh I am torn. I remember him as a three-year-old with those headphones on and listening to the music, man, did he love music. Goodbye David, you will be missed.

It was a warm summer Friday night, July 11, 2003. Denis and I were preparing for an overnight visit to Toronto, leaving the next day. We had tickets to the Lion King on stage, a room booked at a waterfront hotel, and nothing but alone time.

We had been looking forward to this for months. Toronto was still in a recession since 9/11 and they were offering some great package deals to draw people in. It seemed to be working because we bought in.

When the phone rang at 11:30 p.m. that Friday night, I knew it wasn't good news. What worried me was that our younger daughter was still out. The older one was off camping/tubing with friends at Elora Gorge. Those were my two main concerns that fateful night.

It was my sister and she had terrible news. My nephew David, my other sister's twenty-five-year-old son had been killed in a motorcycle accident. A large SUV made an illegal left-hand turn in front of David and he T-boned the SUV. He was killed almost instantly when his handlebars crushed his sternum. He tore his aorta and bled to death. David's live-in girlfriend at the time was a passenger on the bike and she was badly injured. David had gone to pick her up at a bar as she'd had drinks and shouldn't drive. Her injuries were extensive: a broken back, broken ribs, a neck injury, and other abrasions. They couldn't give her anything for pain as her blood alcohol level was too high, so she had to tough out the pain for several hours.

My first reaction when I got the call was, "Are you sure?" Stupid question I know, but likely a common one. I was horrified. I couldn't imagine my sister's agonizing pain. I wanted to get to her right away but when you live two hours away from home, it's not always so simple.

Denis and I decided we'd wait and go down when both girls were home and they could come with us. We wanted to show our support as a solid family. The logistics of us staying somewhere for a few days was not always ideal and we had to put a plan in place.

I waited for the younger one to get home. She snuck in quietly because she thought she was in trouble. We had just spoken to her the night before about her curfew and she was late again. Truthfully, that was the last thing on my mind. I explained to her what happened and that we'd be heading to Stoney Point once we either got in touch with her older sister or when she got home.

We got up after absolutely no sleep and called the campground where the older one was staying as she did not have a cell phone back then. We told the park ranger to please have her call us ASAP as we had a family emergency. They must have gone straight to her as she called within minutes on someone's cell phone. Unfortunately, the phone she was using died right after I told her there'd been a terrible accident, so I didn't get to give her any other information. She experienced an agonizing ten minutes until she got to the desk, explained that she had an emergency, and needed to use a phone. By now, she was sobbing and thought something had happened to her sister. I explained that her cousin David had been in a terrible accident and died as a result. She was horrified because David's sister is a very close cousin and our daughter knew she'd be in terrible pain.

Our oldest was camping with other people and had ridden in their car. We decided to meet at our place on Sunday morning, then we'd head to Stoney Point from there. Denis and I decided to go to Toronto after all and see the show. I was back and forth on that decision as my heart wanted to be with my sister, but I knew what the scene would end up being like and I wanted none of it.

Denis and I drove to Toronto in relative silence with tears streaming down my face most of the ride there. We tried to cheer up but how could we? We checked into the hotel and headed to the show. The show was beautiful: the music, the costumes, all of it was amazing. I won't give it away but there's a scene where they sang *"The Circle of Life"* and I was ugly bawling, I mean tears pouring down my cheeks, snot everywhere kind of crying. Sitting next to me was a little girl of about four years old who was with her mother. She leaned towards me, patted my hand, and said, "Don't worry, they are just acting. He's not really dead." That touched me deeply, for a little child to understand that I was so sad and in her innocence thought it was about the show. How could she possibly grasp the reality I was facing and that particular song was choking me with the irony?

I wasn't crying about the show, I was crying about the loss of my first nephew. I loved that boy. I babysat him as a child, fed him, changed his diapers, played with him, danced with him in my arms, snuck him candy when he wasn't supposed to have it, and we had all kinds of fun together. I was crying because I knew my sister was in pain and I was so far from her. I was crying because all our lives were changed forever. I was crying because I was helpless. I could never take that pain away from my sister. I was crying because, for the rest of her life, she would carry this burden.

To this day, I'm haunted by this decision. Would it have made a difference for me to be there? Would I have been intruding on their private time? Yes, I think I would have, and I wanted to grieve in my own way for just a couple of days.

Once we returned from Toronto and our daughter returned from her camping trip, we all met at home, packed up our bags and headed straight out to my sister's home. We offered our sincerest condolences and didn't stay long as I suspected they'd had plenty of visitors in the last day or two and needed to plan for the funeral.

The funeral was very special – a true memorial to David. They played music David would have loved, including Pink Floyd's *"Wish You Were Here"* and many others. They had a motorcycle procession ahead of the hearse and did a "revving" tribute to him. There had to be least fifty motorcycles revving their motorcycles all at once. It was loud, stirring, and eerily beautiful. For my sister, her husband, and their daughter, I believe it was touching. It would have made David happy for sure.

My nephew was a gifted musician and fought the drug scene in a horrible way. He tried to kick the habit but was hooked fiercely. His family supported him in his sobriety; we all believed that he had licked the problem. When they went to his place after the accident, they found sheet music. This was the last project he had been working on. It makes me happy to know that this was the last thing he did before dying. He loved his music. It was his happy place.

Straight from the funeral, there was a burial and then a luncheon. After that, we all went to my sister's home. David's wishes were to empty his bank account and buy beer to celebrate his life. He had told my sister this once, so they did it. She jokes that there was enough for a six-pack!

Many people shared stories about David and it was poignant. I stood up to tell mine: "When David was about two years old, he called me Aunt Barie, 'M's' were still hard for him. At our older daughter's baptismal, he pointed to the Virgin Mary and yelled out Aunt Barie! Most people didn't get the joke but at her baptismal, I was still unmarried and for him to point to the Virgin Mary and call her Aunt Barie was very funny. Everyone at the party got a good laugh about that as twenty-three years had passed since then, so it was no longer taboo. David loved a good laugh and that is how I choose to remember my nephew." Love you and miss you, Dave. XO

Chapter Nineteen

MEME'S DEATHBED TALE – AUGUST 2003

Dear Diary,

Oh my, I just got off the phone with Mom. She is fit to be tied! I guess Meme lied to her on her deathbed about her birth father. Oh dear. I get that Meme comes from a different generation but really, can she not just tell Mom the truth, does she think Mom would judge her? I couldn't do much but listen, and some days that's all some people need. They just need you to listen, not try to solve anything; just an ahem, ahem here or there and she got to express herself. It was heart breaking to listen to her sad voice.

It was Mom's turn to care for her mother, Meme D. Her brothers and sisters all took turns to go there and stay overnight. They would cook for her, bathe her, help her with her medications, or any other needs Meme had. They took care of it all.

On one particularly warm evening, Mom's son had called to speak to her, but Meme picked up the phone. She spoke to him for a minute or two and then passed the phone to Mom. Once Mom was off the phone, Meme D. told her that he sounded just like Mom's birth father. Mom thought this the most opportune time to ask her one more time about her birth father. In the past when she would ask, she would get reprimanded and told to never bring it up again.

Meme directed Mom to a shoebox with photos in it. In it was a picture of what Mom thought was her little sister but turned out to be her mother, Meme D. She was in high heels wearing bobby socks and was posing with a very good-looking man whom Mom thought looked just like her son. Turns out it was Meme with her boyfriend at the time. Mom thought that they looked so happy.

Meme D. told her of how she worked in the states with her friend. They would go downtown after work for a bowl of soup, listen to the big bands, and dance. Oh, how Meme D. loved to dance. One evening they met this group of fellows from Texas who said they were construction workers. There she met a man they called Dutchy. After this, they'd meet every Thursday for soup and dancing. He tried to talk her into going to his hotel room, but she told him she was a respectable "girl" and couldn't do that unless she was married.

She went on and explained to Mom that the following Thursday he showed up with a minister. They proceeded to his hotel room where they had a ceremony and she stayed with him in his room for three days. After the third day, there was a knock on the door. It was Dutchy's father. He took his son away and told Meme D. to never come back.

Sadly, she told Mom, that is how she got to be pregnant and had no way to reach him. She never heard from him again. It was all very believable to Mom. She so badly wanted to believe the story about her father. At least she had a story about her father now.

A couple of months after Meme D's death, Mom went to visit her aunt, Meme's sister, at a rest home for seniors. She loved her aunt dearly and felt she needed to visit her. Once there and they were settled with their tea, her aunt asked Mom if her mother had finally told her the truth about her father. Mom wisely said, "Oh yes, she did. But I'd love to hear it again from you." Mom just let her Aunt talk and it turned out that Meme D. had lied on her deathbed to her own daughter (Mom) or had she told Mom the truth and not her sister? What is more likely?

Mom's aunt told her about Meme's boyfriend and how they were in love, but Pepe would not let him in after Meme D. got pregnant; he would not allow it. She said that the boyfriend never married, never had children, and would often inquire about Mom, her whereabouts, and how she was. He knew of her marriage to Dad and of her eight children. The truth was that the picture Meme D. had shown Mom was of that boyfriend, her father, and that he had never married.

Shortly after this visit, Mom went to visit her aunt, another sister of Meme D. She brought a dish of lazy man cabbage rolls for her. Her aunt corroborated with her sister on the story and confirmed that indeed the old boyfriend was Mom's father and not Dutchy as her mother had told her on her deathbed. Mom was furious with her mother. Why would she take this secret to her grave? Did she not know how important this was to her?

These questions were difficult for Mom's aunt to answer and the only response she had for Mom was that her sister had been an extremely proud woman. She had vowed to take that secret to her grave and by golly, she did just that.

Today you can do DNA testing, hire a detective, and there's even an app now to find your father. All of these were not available to Mom in her lifetime and that is incredibly sad. I wish she had found out who her real father was when she was younger. Perhaps there was a grandfather out there who wanted to be a part of our lives!

It was one of Mom's only regrets in life that she never found her birth father. If you're looking for a birth parent or you gave a baby up for adoption, be brave and go seek them out! They may have been wondering as all the years pass and those are years you could've spent with them!

You could be unlocking a Pandora's box or you could be opening a treasure chest filled with new experiences, adventures, and celebrations.

You could have sisters, brothers, nieces, nephews, and ***grandchildren*** just waiting to meet you. How can you take the chance that you'd miss out on this? I'll never know my real grandfather and that is so sad. Don't make the mistake my grandmother did.

If you have a child you adopted, isn't it time to be honest with them? Is it fair to hold that info from them? I have two nieces that were adopted and their parents have been honest from day one. I very much respect that. Those nieces are now adults and have met their birth parents. It is their choice if they choose to have a relationship with their birth parents or not. I believe that is the kindest solution.

Chapter Twenty

DAD PASSES – JUNE 2005

Dear Diary,

How do I express how I feel tonight? Am I sad? Yes, I am sad. I'm sad I didn't have a dad as most people have. He never told me he was proud of me, was he? He never told me he loved me, did he? Did he know how to love? Maybe I'm sad that my children got cheated out of a Pepe? Why did he not get the joy, the blessing of children? Does it matter now? I guess not. I remember, not that long ago, we were at our Aunt and Uncle's 50th anniversary party and Mom told Dad she forgave him; he was blown away. I think that's as close to love I've seen him express.

On April 20, 2005, exactly a year after our eldest daughter's wedding in Mexico, I started a new full-time job. The company was a food broker and given that our younger daughter was in University now, a bigger paycheque was coming in handy. Remember me saying I needed to spend less time on the road? Well, that went out the window with this job. I was traveling further and longer than before.

On June 4, 2005, at 8 a.m., I was packing up my car for another day on the road, selling some of my varied lines at the time. I was working and on this day, I was slated to be in the Kitchener area. I had come back into the house for something that I forgot to pack, and the phone was ringing.

I usually would let it go to voicemail, but something told me to answer the phone. It was my sister. She said, "Sit down, I have news." It's never good when they tell you to sit down, is it?

She said that Dad had passed away during the night. He did not suffer, and at this moment, she didn't have any details. He died of natural causes, but they had no funeral plans as of yet. I thought to myself, "This is going to be strange." Relations with Dad's wife and family were awkward at best.

I actually considered going out to work that day but called and spoke with my sales manager and gave him the news. He told me to unpack my samples and to take as much time as I needed. I thought that was odd, but I suppose he had no idea of the relationship I had with my father, or lack thereof. I agreed it was best to stay off the road. It turned out I was right; I was scatterbrained for days.

I called Denis at work and gave him the news. He asked if I was alright and if I wanted him to come home. I said that I'd like to have the day to just chill and think of my dad. He called a few times during the day to check on me but really, I wasn't feeling too sad, just yet. I spoke to a few friends and waited until the end of the day to tell the girls, our daughters. Nothing could be done right now anyhow.

I took the day to ponder on how I felt. I sat in the garden on the big lounge chair, sipping my iced tea, and trying to figure out why I was sad. Was this sadness...or was it regret? I didn't miss him; I knew that. I hadn't seen him in months, and then only once or twice the year prior. We had been on the outs for a long time after Mom and Dad's divorce and had only recently reconciled.

You see, my father was an absentee father. He had different capabilities than most. He just didn't get it. He didn't grasp the joy of being a parent, the day-to-day smiles you get from your kids. We were a pain in the butt to him; at least that's how I felt. I'd like to think that if he were alive today, he would've evolved and that he would get it. I truly believe he was distracted by sex, obsessed even. He was a narcissist, only concerned with his pleasure, his needs at all times.

I could go on and carry a grudge for the rest of my life, as I certainly have felt ripped off in the Daddy Department, but I choose to forgive. I choose to believe that he didn't know any better and if he did, he would have done better.

Eventually, I called our girls and they took the news well. They weren't really surprised and were supportive of me. They both said to keep them in the loop regarding the funeral arrangements and carried on. They hadn't had much to do with their Pepe in a long time and he wasn't actively involved in their lives even when he was around.

The funeral service was in Stoney Point, the town in which Dad grew up in, as did I. There were no visitations, simply a funeral service but many people wanted to pay their respects to us, so my siblings and I formed a line down the aisle of the church and accepted people for quite a while before the service started. Dad's wife, the young waitress, had not made arrangements for us siblings so we ended up being spread throughout the church wherever there was room. I sat rather far back with my family and my in-laws.

My mother sat with a few of the siblings. Yes, my mother came to Dad's funeral even after all the pain and trouble he had caused her. Everyone knows that you don't go to the funeral for the deceased but for the people who lost someone. It was comforting to have Mom and most of my siblings there.

I felt somewhat disrespected due to the lack of reserved seating for us, yet there at the front sat his much younger wife and her two kids. I thought to myself, "That should be us up there. Nevertheless, does it really matter where I sit to send my father off to meet his maker?" My ego was feeling the sting, but was it really that important?

As I sat in the pew with my family, and while the priest was praying/speaking, my mind drifted. Memories flooded my brain like a recap playing on TV. I saw a little girl sitting on her daddy's lap reading a storybook. Was that a memory or a wish? I saw the snowmobile go into the water, soaking my little brother and I. Dad fed us Cherry Whiskey to ward off pneumonia and warned us to never tell Mom. I saw Dad doing doughnuts in parking lots to scare us half to death, doing more doughnuts on icy, snowy roads, laughing his fool head off. Was this his way of being a father? Did he think scaring us was a way to show love? I believe he did.

I saw myself being walked down the aisle, shaking with nervous energy in anticipation that he'd tell me he loved me, hoping that would be the one time he'd say it...but, alas, it did not happen. It just wasn't in him to be vulnerable or to express feelings to his children.

I saw a younger Dad building things with his boys, or as he'd call them, "the little bastards." There was a hammer in one hand, a pencil over his ear, and an apron full of nails, all ready to go.

I saw the frail man that he'd become due to Parkinson's disease, in his last days, weeks, and months when I'd bring cookie samples and how he'd call me Seven (I was born seventh). He would have hated how frail he'd become; he had always said he'd never get old.

I sat with tears of what could have been, should have been, but not so much of missing him, as most people who saw my tears were likely led to think. I hadn't missed him for a long time as he was never really present in my life or that of my siblings. I don't say this to be heartless, it was just our reality.

Following the service, we all headed out into the cool, breezy day to bury Dad's ashes in the cemetery right next to my nephew David's plot. On the way to the burial, my sister was walking along, and our brother told her to stop walking and look at her shoulder. There sat a blue dragonfly for the longest of times. She was certain it was her son David, as did most of us. He stuck around for the service like a good grandson would have. Thanks Dave, you made your mother's day that day.

After the cemetery formalities, a luncheon was served in the church basement. My mother, the seven siblings, and our families all attended. There was mostly family present but that was still likely close to a hundred people, if not more. Dad came from a large family, most of whom had many children plus our family is quite large as well. There was the usual food at funeral luncheons, such as sandwiches, salads, deviled eggs, but best of all was the "tartes au sucre" (sugar pie) which I assume one of the aunts brought along. Many of the family members would come to our table where we all sat and offered their sympathies, which were kindly welcomed.

At the table, my brother shared with us Dad's last meaningful words to him. "Everything changed between your mother and me the day you were born," he went on. "Dad was many things, some bad, and some good but if he was anything at all, he was weak in character. Something I have always strived not to be." Rest in peace Dad, I love you and I forgive you.

Chapter Twenty-One

AUNT SUSIE'S FAILING HEALTH – 2010

Dear Diary,

Today we laid Aunt Susie to rest. She didn't have an easy life, molested as a little girl, then by my father. Plus, she was forced to break up with her fiancée, forced to have her tubes tied at 27, never to have children of her own, then was dumped the minute she aged. She had a hard life. May she Rest in Peace knowing she's been forgiven the mistakes that she made, too weak to do better.

My Aunt and Uncle held a family Christmas brunch every year on Christmas morning, to which the whole family was invited. Some years they had more people attend than other years, depending on availability. During the Christmas holidays of 2010, I asked Mom about her family breakfast, who had attended, what they served for breakfast, etc. She told me that she had seen Aunt Susie who was complaining of a very sore belly. Mom said that her belly looked big or swollen. I didn't think much of it at the time but a couple of months later, on one of our Sunday morning chats, Mom told me that Aunt Susie had cancer. Mom was rather naïve when it came to medical knowledge and said it was cancer of the belly button. I did my own research.

Aunt Susie, my roommate for years and my father's dirty little secret, had been diagnosed with Sister Mary Joseph Nodule. This is a malignant tumor in the abdomen. The nodule is a hard mass bulging into the belly button which is associated with a metastasizing intra-abdominal cancer. It usually indicates a poor prognosis according to my research. In this case, Dr. Google wasn't so far off.

Aunt Susie was taken to London, Ontario to see a specialist and they did a full hysterectomy as her ovaries were full of cancer, not to mention the Sister Mary Joseph Nodule. She would have chemo and a long battle ahead of her. She was in complete denial of her prognosis, believing she could beat it. I wish it were true.

Five years earlier she'd had unusual vaginal bleeding. Had her doctor at that time looked and tested further, perhaps they would have caught the cancer at an earlier stage. Who can say really?

In the fall of 2013, Mom received a phone call from Aunt Susie. She was furious with Mom because their younger brother had told Aunt Susie that he'd been talking with someone and he had the impression that Mom was telling her kids that Aunt Susie was dying. She ranted and raved at Mom, with the "how dare you" and "I am not dying." The rant went on and on. Mom was very hurt that Aunt Sue would lash out at her without giving her a chance to explain, but she let her off the hook again, which left Aunt Susie feeling like everything was fine. It wasn't... Mom was feeling stung.

At the end of July of 2015, Aunt Susie was taken to the hospice where she breathed her last breath. Mom, thinking she was releasing Aunt Susie, again forgave her and told her to go in peace. Mom then left her while her sister-in-law who stayed by Aunt Susie's side. She died on July 28, 2015.

I accompanied Mom to the funeral for Aunt Susie, along with my brother and my sister. Some people have asked me why I would go to her funeral after all she had done to Mom and our family. I answered this quite honestly by saying that Aunt Susie was very good to me. I loved her despite her faults and will leave the judging to God! I had forgiven Aunt Susie a long time ago.

Her funeral was held at a church in Belle River, her hometown. I sat beside Mom in the pew, my brother and sister to my left. The service was your average funeral service and my cousin did a lovely eulogy. It was touching as he spoke of how supportive and kind Aunt Susie had been. She had been a very generous lady, always thinking of others. Those things were all true.

The weird part came when the priest did his eulogy. When he started going on about what a Christian woman Aunt Susie was, my mother gasped, I mean audibly gasped. The three of us sitting in the pew with her turned to see if she was okay. The more that priest spoke, the angrier she got. I could see that she was visibly fuming. That priest could have said Aunt Susie was a generous woman, she was kind, etc. and it would've been true but to say she was a Christian woman who followed the Ten Commandments was a bit of overkill. He obviously knew nothing of Aunt Susie's past and was orating a canned eulogy that he pulled out whenever he didn't know the deceased.

Upon termination of the service, the family followed the priest out, at which point Mom stated she was not going to the funeral luncheon and didn't even want to walk out with the family. She was furious and was afraid she'd say the wrong things if she faced any one of them. It was probably a good call! Truly, I don't think any of them noticed as we turned and walked out the side door, rather than follow the procession.

From there, we went to my sister's place and had a nice lunch. We had an interesting chat regarding Aunt Susie ourselves. She was a good woman, even though she did some things that she was not proud of, and likely didn't handle well, but nobody deserves to die of cancer. It's a nasty disease. We all agreed, and I don't believe we ever discussed it again.

Rest in peace Aunt Susie. I miss you and love you.

Chapter Twenty-Two

DRAMA IN AUSTRALIA – 2012

August 11, 2011

Dear Diary,

Today I met my first client as a caregiver. She seems like such a nice lady, her smoking might be an issue but first things first. Oh and she asked me to escort her to Australia to visit her son and his family. I mean, how bad can it go?

Dear Diary,

First, I can't believe I'm in Australia! You cannot believe how hot it is. Whoa! Don't get me wrong, I am very grateful for this trip, but this lady is out of her mind. I truly believe the drink brings on paranoia. She had me terrified, she was raging, had something in her hand, ready to attack me. I'm not sure how I calmed her down, but she's gone back to her cottage. Me wanting to steal her family, are you kidding me? As if I don't have enough family! Between Denis and I, we have 16 siblings, not to mention hundreds of cousins, a bazillion aunts and uncles. Really! But we can never have enough friends and that's what these people are, true blue friends. So tomorrow I will go and play with kangaroos, koalas, and whatever else this park promises. Goodnight Diary.... It's been quite a day...

In the spring of 2012, I was looking for work. My sister, who had been a caregiver for fifteen years told me that I should be doing the same as her. She said, "You're caring, you look after people every day, you could do this, and you'd do it well." I gave it some thought and decided that I would give it a go. London is a good-sized city and there are many aged people who don't have a family to support them, to help them do the little things that they can't do anymore. I started spreading the word around that if anybody needed a caregiver, to give me a call.

My friend talked to me about a neighbor of hers who was a bit grumpy, but she needed help and was willing to pay for it. My information was passed on and that evening I got a call from the potential client. We decided to get together.

I met this woman for the first time at her home. We had tea, sat in her backyard at her picnic table, and she smoked...and smoked...and smoked. Not a good sign but I needed the work, so I looked past it. Why do we skim over our instincts? It never goes well when you do.

She asked me what kind of tasks I'd do, and I told her I'd take care of the shopping, errands, tidying her house, laundry, cooking, etc. She loved the idea. She asked me if I'd be a travel companion to Australia. I said I would, but she'd have to pay my expenses, travel, and lodging. She talked of a trip to visit her son in Australia come winter. I told her if she wanted me to do that, I'd go along to help her out.

We hit it off and I started working for her the following week. At first I was doing errands, cleaning, and cooking, but eventually, she had me coming full-time to work in her office along with the household chores. I totally organized her office and her home. I felt we were getting along great and she was telling people that I was the best thing since sliced bread.

When fall arrived, she started talking more and more about the Australian trip. We started planning and she had me researching hotels, etc. I found it odd that we weren't staying with her son as she kept going on about how huge his house was. As well, around this same time, I started to notice signs of excessive drinking, but again, I turned a blind eye. I'm telling you; it never ends well when you enter the denial zone.

As Christmas neared, the trip was booked, flights booked, hotels booked, and communications kept flowing back and forth with the son and daughter-in-law. It felt awkward at first which is odd for me; normally I hit it right off with people, but I felt something and I couldn't quite put my finger on it. Again, I ignored my feelings...why didn't I ask more questions?

At Christmas, my client and I exchanged gifts. I wished her a merry holiday and I took a week off to spend time with my family. When I returned seven days later, her recycle bin was filled to the top with liquor bottles. I sprained my back lifting the bin, trying to get it to the road for pick-up. Ugh, only five days until the start of a very long trip to Australia. I needed my chiropractor and fast, plus a few days to rest my back but she saw this as me taking more time off and made sure I knew that she was not impressed.

My chiropractor treated me almost daily. He even came in on a Sunday morning to treat me and by Wednesday I was ready for flying. In my eyes, it was a small miracle. I thought my back would not ever be better. Five days previous, I hadn't been able to stand straight, let alone sit on a plane for way too many hours.

We had a five-hour flight to LAX, and from there we flew to Australia which was another twelve-hour flight. When we landed in Sydney, we missed our flight to Adelaide due to my slow-moving client. She was missing her drink, but I had no idea how much! We soon caught the next flight. We were greeted by her son and I immediately felt the strain between them. There were no big hugs, or I've missed you, and that's when I started to clue in that perhaps this was not just a visit to her son's. It was about time that I caught on!

He took the scenic route to our cottages and for that I was grateful. He was very polite to me, but I found him a bit cool with his mother, whom he called by her given name. Interesting, I thought. She was in a big hurry to get to the liquor store and sent me in to get her vermouth. They did not have her brand and she was not happy about that. I reminded her we were in a different country and perhaps she could make do with the one I bought for her. I held back on the "or go get it yourself" comment.

After driving on the beach and making our way to our cottages, her son dropped us off with the promise of dinner in a couple of hours. We had time to shower, unpack, and get ready so we could go see her grandkids and her daughter-in-law. I helped her unpack and got her settled, and then off we went to their family home. We did, in fact, have a delicious meal of lamb, potatoes, vegetables, as well as a lovely watermelon salad – it was my favorite thing that night.

Our first day there she was on her best behavior, bringing gifts for her grandkids, watching her language, being careful not to swear in front of them, being nice to her daughter-in-law; and she'd only had only one glass of wine.

I was trying my utmost to be helpful to our hosts, helping with the cooking, dishes, and the children. They were preparing some delicious meals for us and frankly my client was not being very gracious. One day, she asked her daughter-in-law when she was going to make her a good meal because we'd only had junk so far. I was appalled and told her to pipe down; everything we'd had so far was wonderful. I was a bit shocked by her behavior but until this trip, I'd only had to endure her for a few hours at a time and she was usually well-behaved. But now, having spent many hours in her company, I was finding it interesting to discover how she behaved without alcohol, or at least not at her normal consumption level; it was obviously starting to have an effect on her. She was getting grumpier by the second.

On the third day there, her daughter-in-law said she'd take me for a driving lesson so that I could borrow the car to take the client and her grandkids to the beach or do some touring. Her son was to spend some time with his mother and the grandkids, and I was totally oblivious to the fact that my client was paranoid about me spending time alone with her daughter-in-law. I mean ***paranoid***.

So off we went for a drive on the right-handed side lesson. We stopped for coffee/tea and lunch and had a great get-to-know each other kind of visit. I spoke of my family and she spoke of hers. I touched on my client and her son's relationship and asked a bit about that. It turns out that she and her son hadn't spoken in several years and this was their reunion of sorts. She didn't go into much detail, and I didn't dare to ask just yet.

That night the client wanted to get back to the cottage early, so her son took her back. The daughter-in-law and I went back out for another driving lesson. She took me to the beach and we saw an amazing Australian sunset! When we returned from the driving lesson, we all had a glass of wine and just socialized.

Around 11 o'clock that evening, her son drove me back to my cottage and I started to get ready for bed. I was in the bathroom, brushing my teeth, and all at once there was pounding on my door and bedroom window. I was frightened at first as it was pitch black in this area at night and I didn't know nary a soul. Then I heard the voice. It was my client and she was angry. But why would she be angry with me?

I could smell the alcohol on her as soon as I opened the door, and then the shouting started followed by accusations. She was afraid that I was stealing her family from her. Really? Have I mentioned that I have seven siblings? I don't need more family, thank you very much. She actually frightened me, and I told her in a very firm voice to go to bed, get some rest, and that we'd discuss it tomorrow. She fired me at that very moment and I again said we'd discuss it tomorrow.

The next day the daughter-in-law and the kids picked us up to go to Urimberra, a nature reserve where I was promised I'd see many kangaroos. I couldn't wait! I mean real live kangaroos, where I could touch them, come on! My client was in a sour mood from the start. She was dressed in heels and her daughter-in-law told her that there was unsteady ground and that she may be more comfortable in a flat shoe. But no! She decided to be stubborn and wore the heels. We all applied sunscreen on as it was high noon and the sun gets scorchingly hot in Australia, but she flatly refused to. All day she was snipping at me, but I ignored it and let it go. She fired me again that day and at that point, I'd had enough of her abuse and gladly accepted that she fired me.

The next evening, she had plans with her "army vet" friends whom she had met online. They were getting together for some social time, so her daughter-in-law had invited me to a scrapbooking evening with her friend. They taught me how to do a scrapbook page and I did a pretty good job. I was impressed, though all accolades went to them.

On the way back to my cottage, she asked me about the day before and her mother-in-law had been so snarky all day. I filled her in on the happenings of the night prior and she was horrified for me. This behavior is exactly why they'd had no contact with her for so long. I was sad. I didn't want to cause trouble for anybody especially this wonderful family.

The next day, the daughter-in-law and son came to pick us up and told my client she would have to play nice and be civil or she'd not be allowed in their home. They wanted peace and harmony in their home, not her shouting or cursing. My client told them it was her or me, and that she had no intention of being nice to me. They said, "Fine, we choose her!" They came to my cottage, told me to grab my purse, and we pulled out of there like the car was on fire. We were practically on two wheels when we zoomed out of there. She was on her porch swearing at us, shaking her fist, throwing things. It felt as if I was in a soap opera! We went back later that evening to pick up my things and emptied my cottage while she was out with her friends. I didn't see her for the rest of the trip, and I was grateful for that.

I spent the rest of my "holiday" with the family. They were amazing hosts and were so very kind. I called the airline and paid extra to have my ticket changed so that I could get home a day earlier than expected to avoid traveling with my client. Also, it would allow me to get home earlier to visit Fred in the hospital, or so I thought.

While I was in Australia, I used Skype to talk with Denis and I also phoned home a couple of times. On one such internet call, which was Sunday morning for me and Saturday evening for Denis, he was telling me about his visit with Fred and how sick Fred was. He had also taken Mom home as she had felt ill at the hospital. He stayed with her until my brother arrived. Denis had a very long day while I was sleeping in Australia.

We were still talking online when his phone rang. He looked at me inquiringly, and I said, "Go ahead, answer it." It was my brother-in-law calling to tell Denis that Fred had passed away. I hadn't realized the severity of things and now I wouldn't get a chance to say goodbye. I was very sad and to be so far from home at a time like this was very hard. I wasn't there for my mother, for my family, and it was breaking my heart into pieces.

I tried reaching Mom but when I called, I was told she was sleeping. She had been completely exhausted by the weeks of Fred being in the hospital and it was taking a toll. Today we know that she likely was already sick, but we just didn't know it yet. I would not get to speak to her till I got home on Wednesday.

The family decided to have the funeral for Fred on Wednesday, so I was unable to attend. I honestly thought they would wait for me for the funeral, as it would've been one more day to wait. I was broken-hearted that I wasn't important enough for them to wait one stinking day. I wanted to be there for Mom and my siblings; to say my farewells to Fred.

I left Australia on Tuesday morning. For me to attend the funeral, I would've had to leave on Monday morning, but I didn't know till Monday afternoon when the funeral was.

Early Tuesday morning my client's son took me to the airport and sat with me while I waited for my flight. I had left notes for each of the kids, for him and his wife which they would read after I left. I had poured my heart out in the letters, and I felt I had met lifetime friends over the most unusual circumstances.

My flight was long and quiet which gave me time to reflect on things, to quietly say goodbye to Fred, and to go over my holiday. My client still had no idea that I had changed my flight. She would be pretty ticked when she found out.

She tried suing me for $25,000, stating that I did not care for her while on the holiday. The case was sided in my favor after months of court dates. Not only had she fired me several times, but I had witnesses who heard her say that this was a holiday and not a work trip. She was very abusive to me while in Australia and threatened me with violence. The drama was over, the judge sided with me. Phew! The judge told her that he was sorry we hadn't been able to work it out and he felt that she had lost a very attentive caregiver. I would never see her again.

Chapter Twenty-Three

PARENTING ADVICE

Dear Diary,

This morning I got a call from a frantic my older daughter. She's on her way to work and her little guy is vomiting! She feels she can't take another day off, and since today is my day off, could I watch the kids? Of course, I said yes. And she's on her way. She arrives, with both kids covered in vomit, as well as her back seat and car seats covered in it ... she's near tears, and I tell her to clean up the car and hand me the baby. "Sweetie, come with Meme, you're gonna play in the bathtub!" Poor little guy has a bug, and the smell had his sister gagging first, then vomiting! Thank goodness she wasn't sick too. I mean, I'm good but not that good! She "washed" up in the tub while I cleaned her little brother, then settled him in the crib. We got through the day. My daughter cleaned the car the best she could and headed to work. Today when we talk about it, she wonders why she didn't just go home. I tell her that it was because she had just gotten back to work and felt obligated to go. It's OK! It's a difficult balance being a working mom. "You got this." I said. Parenting doesn't end at 18, just saying!

Mom and I had many discussions regarding parenting. Talking to Mom about raising kids was like discussing religion with the Pope. It could go on for hours and hours. Was she a perfect mother? It depends on who you asked. Is there such a thing as a perfect parent? I don't think so. We're all human, we all do or say things we regret, it happens.

I asked her one day if it was easier to parent girls or boys. Her reply was that, depending on the different stages, both are easier or harder. Well, that was clear as mud! She clarified by saying perhaps boys were harder when they're small because they just want to run wild, while girls might be tougher to deal with when they are teenagers and their hormones are raging.

What we both agreed on was that our children are affected by where we are in life. As an example, I was a working mom to my elder daughter. She was in daycare and I was at work, which was our normal. Today, she is a working mom herself. Did I, as a working mom, shape her future? To further prove my point, I was a stay-at-home mom while my youngest daughter was growing up. Today, she is a stay-at-home mom. Again, did my being home affect her future differently? As a parent, I believe that as you are learning and growing, depending on the birth order, the children will be affected or shaped differently.

Another parenting tip Mom and I agreed on was that not enough parents use the ***"no!"*** It's only a couple of letters but too many children are growing up to be entitled because they've never been told "no." It's totally acceptable to occasionally just say "no." We don't have to give our children every little thing they want or agree to every party, trip, or event they want to go to. They will be okay. When the girls got older, we had a rule with them. We would buy everything that they needed, and they would buy what they wanted. It's funny, when they put out their own money how differently their purchases look.

Remember when your children were small, and you thought changing dirty diapers all day was hard? Well, have you seen a mother on the first day of school about to load her precious cargo onto a big yellow tin can to let them go into the world all on their own? Now that is tough. Then there are the teen years. They'll knock those younger years out of the ballpark in a minute, won't they? I think that's why babies are so cute. By the time they're teens, you already really love them, and you think they can do no wrong. That is until they hit PMS...Goodness! It's not fair for parents or these poor teen girls to go through that. I think if we'd had a better understanding that these young girls were going through a huge hormonal stage. they're frightened by it as much as we are, and we give them a bit of space, then life would be a bit easier for everyone.

Then the dating starts. Are we ever ready for this? I can recall a few boys coming in to meet us and shaking in their boots. One young lad, who shall remain nameless, was just sweating bullets. His forehead was covered in beads of sweat, his cheeks were rosy, and his mouth dry as cotton balls. I have to say from a parent's point of view, I got a bit of disturbed enjoyment out of his discomfort. I always reminded them on the way out the door to drive safely and to remember that was my daughter they were driving around with, not just their girlfriend. "I went through many hours of labor for her and if anything happens to her, her big and strong father will be the least of your worries!" I would say this with the slightest smile, like the Cheshire cat just before he swallows the canary.

I had a friend who asked me if I had any tricks or clues because her daughter was starting to date, and I told her that I had one thing for her to do. "Okay, what's that?" she asked. "Make beans whenever she is going on a date," I replied. "Beans?" she asked. "Yes ma'am, think about it...what do beans do to you. If you serve them right before they're heading out, then about one to two hours later, the effects will kick in. Trust me, she'll want to get home soon and won't be getting too comfortable with any boy!" My daughter says I'm crazy if I think that helped at all! I'm sticking to my story. Make beans!

I joke but seriously though, you need to talk to your daughters ***and*** sons regarding protection. Not only do they need to worry about STD's, but there are unplanned pregnancies to think of too.

You get through the teens and then they're adults. You get this crazy thought that parenting ends once the girls moved out on their own or got married but surprisingly it doesn't. It just changes. I must admit, I am happy about that. You no longer control their eating habits and hope they'll continue to make proper meals, get a good night's sleep, and lead decent lives. Of course, they do because they remember all that they've learned over the years. Phew!

One of my happiest days as a mother was when our elder daughter announced her pregnancy. It was very simple how they did it. We were all sitting around the living room having a discussion of some kind and suddenly her husband said, "Well, we have some news to share with you." My first thought was that he had aced a test at school or maybe they got a new car, but no, she said, "We're having a baby in April!" I looked at her and said, "You'd better not be kidding because I will cry," and she said she wasn't! I yelled out a whoop, cried tears while hugs went all around with congratulations. It was a magical moment for everyone! I don't know why I was shocked as they'd been married three years and it was time, but I was so excited that I ran out the door, straight across the street to my friend's house, and had to tell them. Our first precious grandchild came into our world on April 26, 2007, and our world has forever changed. She is a precious miracle for which I will always be grateful to God.

Somehow hearing that our other daughter was pregnant only two years later was still just as magical and even more of a surprise. She called me one day from work. She and her husband had been married only six months now and she was wondering what we were doing on Thursday. I said we're not doing much and invited them to come for dinner. I didn't find this unusual as Denis and I were still getting used to being empty nesters. When the kids call and want to come over for dinner, it was always a good thing and it still is. She said they'd be over after work. Nothing unusual there. We were having a very normal dinner: chicken, her favorite salad with my homemade Italian dressing, mashed potatoes, and green beans. As I was sticking some beans in my mouth, she said that they had news. Me being the innocent one was thinking, "Oh they're moving, or she has a new job."

Nope! They're pregnant! She said they're going to have a baby in late June. Well, blow me over with a feather. We were ecstatic and again hugs and congratulations went all around. I got on the phone and we called her sister right away. As a mother, it is heartwarming to see your two daughters sharing big news like this with each other. I just sat, watched the conversation, and smiled as it wasn't very long ago that I worried they'd never stop bickering.

So, for you parents out there with young children, trust me, it gets better and easier. There are challenges still as they age, and usually, you're simply a sounding board.

Parenting is a lifelong job and the benefits far outweigh the challenges. I genuinely enjoy seeing my daughters now as mothers and hearing them using my lines! I wonder if they even notice they are doing it.

Grandparenting. Now that's a fun job and I plan to milk it for all it's worth. There is nothing like a child saying she loves to come to your house, or can we make more cookies for Pepe? I say bring them on girls!

Each of the girls went on to have one more child. We have a grandson by the eldest daughter and another girl for the youngest daughter. In total, we have four grandkids to spoil and it is our pleasure, to be sure.

Having grandkids is like a second chance at parenting, but they go home eventually. Usually, they are cute, adorable, and funny while here and save all the less than fun stuff for their parents. No wonder my mother enjoyed her grandkids so much.

To relieve their parents, we occasionally host cousin parties. This is a party where the four cousins get together at our place, sans parents. We eat all the right foods, you know – pizza, hot dogs, chicken strips, or nachos. It's easy, why argue? They love it as do we! They like to assemble their own food, so we often do build your own tacos, pizza, or nachos. They love cooking, these kids.

We've been known to have NERF wars, hikes in the woods, sledding, Geocaching, baking, crafting of all kinds, and let's not forget the swimming. They love that pool.

Chapter Twenty-Four

MOM IS OUR GLUE – SPRING 2015

September 28, 2015

Dear Diary,

Today we got news Mom is sick. One sister says she could live ten years and the realistic one says we'll be lucky to get a year with her. I wanna believe I have her for ten but I know that's not possible, Mom is sick already. Dear diary, I'll probably be writing lots as I feel like we're in for a ride with this family. I feel a storm a coming, batten down the hatches.

Dear Diary,

No, no, no, not Mom. I am not ready to let go of Mom. Oh my, she's so sick. Today on my way to visit her I drove all the way to Tecumseh on the 401, missing my turn-off by two or three exits! I was crying like crazy and was very distracted. Not good! Ugh, I just want Mom to be better, but she won't get better. She's in terrible pain, suffering. Oh Mom, Mommy, don't leave me, I need you. Our family is falling apart, you are our glue.

On one of our Sunday morning phone calls, Mom was telling me about her trip to the market in Windsor. She said, "I was going through the checkout paying for my groceries and out of nowhere I vomited, without notice, just hurled all over the place. It was as if someone pushed a button on my back to vomit. It just happened." She was horrified, embarrassed, and not feeling well at all. She had been complaining for months that she wasn't feeling well but her doctor kept telling her that she had the flu or a virus. This was an obvious case of ageism. I spoke with my sister and asked her to accompany Mom to the doctor and not take no for an answer. The doctor ***had*** to send her for blood work or send her to a specialist!

My sister went with Mom to the doctor in August 2015 because she had shortness of breath. He told her he was sending her to a heart specialist, in Chatham, who turned out to be an internist, a geriatrician internist and had blood work and an X-ray ordered for Mom.

The doctor said the blood showed a certain protein you would find in cancer patients, so he suggested a bone marrow biopsy to confirm it. My sister took Mom to this appointment, made sure Mom was comfortable for this procedure and had them give Mom a "relaxant." It turned out not to be as painful as expected, but that could have been the drugs working.

Then the doctor called my sister and said to bring Mom in; it wasn't good news. My two older sisters took Mom to see him. It was the day after Mom's birthday. He explained to Mom that she had multiple myeloma and leukemia. She asked what the outlook was, and he explained that some people would live up to ten years with treatment. He then continued to explain that it would also depend on many things, like how long she'd had it, her age, her health, and her fitness. She was not fit, she was eighty-one years old, and her health was failing. She most certainly did not have ten years to live.

Mom was referred to an oncologist in Windsor who gave her the treatment plan which Mom followed to a tee. She went to the oncologist every six weeks where they would evaluate her progress and set up the next steps of treatments.

He booked her for her first chemo treatment and Mom was such a trooper. She did not complain one bit. She knew all her eight children supported any and every decision she made. She went for treatments for five weeks then had a week off. The chemo seemed to help at first because her numbers looked good, but the side effects were getting worse each time.

Mom was in treatments until the middle of March 2016 and was then taken by my sister for her follow-up appointment with the doctor in Windsor. He told Mom they were stopping the chemo injections and gave her a choice of either the chemo pill with prednisone, which would extend her life by six months with many side effects or they could stop all treatments so she could live a better quality of life – but a shorter one.

My sister asked how long Mom would live with the chemo combo and the doctor answered that it would be a maximum of one year. Then she asked how much time Mom would have with no treatment and the doctor just tilted her head and didn't answer. So, my sister asked if she was talking six months and this time the doctor shook her head "no." "Four months?" my sister asked. The doctor tilted her head back and forth, which my sister took to mean it was a possibility. This latest diagnosis brought on sadness but no shock to anyone. We had all taken turns bringing Mom to chemo and could see the degradation weekly.

On December 22, 2015, Mom was found blacked out on her floor. She had passed out, been ill, and was lying on the floor in a mess. The ambulance was called, and Mom never went home again. The doctors said she'd need to either have supervision or move into a nursing home.

My sister graciously offered her home and took care of Mom for a full month until her spot at a retirement home was ready. She took great care of Mom, nourishing her, if not willing her, to life again. My sister would tell me how weak Mom was and how hard of a time she had just getting to the toilet. It was so sad for Mom, but my sister cared for her with all her heart. For this, I will be forever grateful to her. She did what none of her seven siblings could or would do.

In January of 2016, Mom moved into a retirement home. At first, she loved it as she was still able to participate in bingo and other activities they had. It was a beautiful facility and she was comfortable.

In the month of March, late one night, Mom was headed to the washroom using her walker when she stumbled. She went flying into the door, shoulder first, and broke her arm right at the shoulder. The poor woman lied in pain for quite a while before she was found by a night nurse. Although the retirement residence is a beautiful place for seniors, it's not a place for the sick. Mom was taken to the hospital by ambulance where they performed X-rays on her arm and her hip. Nobody thought to look at her back even though she complained of back pain...***a lot!***

Two days later I went to visit her. She complained of being in great pain and wanted to go to her bed. My sister, who is a professional caregiver, was there as well. As we assisted Mom to her bed, she was crying out in pain. I went to the desk, asked for the nurse, told her that my mom was crying in pain, and she said, "Well, she's had her meds and I'd need to call the doctor to give her more." I replied that I was okay with that. "Go ahead and call him, even if it is Sunday!" Sometimes you just have to fight for your mother.

Life was getting complicated with our family. There was a lot of "he said, she said" going on regarding Mom's care. When you have seven siblings it can get a bit crazy.

On one of my visits with Mom, I brought her a bowl of tomato macaroni soup, her favorite those days. She loved it! It's the little things people appreciate. So, we were having soup and Mom was telling me that she had raw skin under her breast. She proceeded to lift her shirt to show me, an image I won't soon get out of my head. Who needs to see their mom's breasts? She was right though. It was all chafed and I told her that she needed to dry the area well when she bathed. We'd discuss this with the CCAC ladies who helped her to bathe. She asked me to stay for her doctor's appointment that day, as they had a doctor that visited her once a week and today was that day.

I agreed to stay but I knew it'd be awkward as I had emailed my sister in frustration and said more than I should have. I had insulted and hurt her feelings. I regret doing that and wish I had called her in person. The great thing about e-mail is that no one can interrupt you, which is a real problem in my family.

When my sister arrived, I talked to her about Mom's rash and said maybe we could talk to the night nurses who bathed Mom. Perhaps we should get a baby powder that they could sprinkle under her breasts afterward. "Let's just make her comfortable," I said. My sister didn't like the idea of baby powder and thought the nurses wouldn't do it.

Alas, the doctor arrived and he was talking with Mom. She started to tell him about her rash and without notice, Mom just lifted her top and bared all. Goodness! He agreed that she indeed was chafed. I piped up and asked about the baby powder idea. The doctor liked the suggestion and said he'd start with cortisone cream, then she should add baby powder into her evening bath routine. I thanked him and let him move on to the next patient.

I was so glad that I had stayed and talked to the doctor for Mom. I'm certain my sister could've handled that little bit but for some reason, Mom wanted me there, so I stayed. I didn't get to do much for Mom during her illness so assisting with this little itty-bitty detail made me feel like I somehow helped.

If there's a lesson here, I guess it'd be that if you have siblings and they show a need or want to help in their parent's care, allow them that gift. It's all part of our grieving process and who wouldn't want extra help?

Chapter Twenty-Five

FORGIVENESS

Dear Diary,

Today I had my standing Sunday call with Mom; let's be real, how many more will I have with her? What will I do every Sunday morning? Her sitting there with her coffee, and me with my tea, the two of us just chatting. Today we talked about forgiveness, her favourite topic. She said one of my siblings was ticked off about something I pinned on Faceplate (her words). She says what the Hell is that anyway? I said well Mom, it's like a digital bulletin board where you pin things on, pictures, sayings, etc. We call it Facebook. But the kicker is, everyone that's a friend can see it. Sometimes you put something up and people get offended. I said, "Do you know what I think Mom?" She says, "What ya got?" I replied to Mom, "I think we post things we need to be reminded of, but someone may see it and read into it, thinking it's about them, it may be a big flashing sign from above saying maybe they should look inward. Mom, whoever it is, just tell them I love them no matter what. I never said I was perfect."

In many of my conversations with Mom, while she was at the Retirement Home, she spoke of forgiveness. She told me it's most important to forgive people as it lightens the heart. We all have different meanings or ways around forgiveness. For me, it means to let go of the anger, bitterness, frustration, vulnerability, and resentment for an action that was hurtful to me. That person may not even know they are hurting you – completely oblivious – and here you are holding on to all this negativity. Let it go; it's unhealthy. Some people waste their entire lives and even go to their graves not forgiving people. Is it really worth carrying that burden all of your life?

I asked Mom, "But how do you forgive people Mom? There are people who've really hurt my feelings and I think it's unforgivable the way that some people behaved. How do I forgive them?" Her reply was simply "You just do. You say 'I forgive you,' and that's it, Marie, it's not rocket science!" To which she added, "Bake them the lemon cupcakes!" I said, "Whaaat...those were forgiveness cupcakes all those years?" She replied, "Maybe." Nothing says love like a lemon cupcake! Wow, just wow...I had no idea. I can't tell you how many times I came home from school and there were lemon cupcakes on the counter, ready to be nibbled on! I wonder who she was forgiving all those times because we ate a lot of lemon cupcakes over the years.

I did a bit of my own research as the cupcakes weren't cutting it for me. It turns out that forgiveness is a change in the way you think. The key is to release suffering and increase inner peace and understanding. Forgiveness is ***not*** overlooking the people who wronged you. Forgiveness is ***not*** forgetting or saying that something will be treated as acceptable behavior in the future. Forgiveness is, first and foremost, done for the person doing the forgiving. Forgiveness is your way to freedom. It frees you from the control of the person who caused the harm. They lose their power to cause you to feel negative emotions. Forgiveness can break old patterns that might otherwise impede when you try to create new relationships. Forgiveness can take a lot of time and industriousness.

Forgiveness need not require working it out with the person who caused the harm. It is an internal process and is primarily for you. The goal is to help you heal and to help you grow. Thinking about forgiveness may not be enough. Meditation, interpersonal dialogues, and intense emotional work may be essential parts of the forgiveness process for many people.

Many people take vitamins for their immune systems, but what about feeding their souls' immune systems? Feed it love, forgiveness, acceptance, gratitude, kindness, and just let go of the other negativity. I think it's all a bit more complicated than what Mom says, but the bottom line is to forgive the offense and then stop going on about it. You're boring the poor people who have to listen to you! Instead, talk about the things you are grateful for. Don't give the bitterness any air – don't fan it. Just keep living day by day, and eventually, you'll be able to say "It happened, it was unpleasant, I'm not proud of how I handled it, but today I can do better. I do not claim to be perfect, far from it, for the record...nobody is." I've done things that I'm not proud of during Mom's illness and have apologized to those I offended. If they choose to forgive, that's up to them.

Surprisingly, Mom forgave her sister who had an affair with her husband for almost thirty years. Mom forgave Aunt Susie shortly after Mom and Dad divorced. On her sister's deathbed, Mom told Aunt Susie not to worry about the affair, she was forgiven, and she could go in peace. Mom said, "Go and be happy. Don't worry, I had forgiven you a long time ago." Her sister died just hours after this, so Mom believes it lightened her heart.

I, too, forgave my aunt. I truly believe that she did the best she could with what she was given in life. Could she have done things differently? Sure, but truly, who are we to judge? There are some people who cannot forgive, and that's okay. I forgive them and that's going to have to be enough until they're ready. We're not all in the same lane, let alone on the same highway!

Mom also forgave Dad. He was not a very good husband and perhaps a worse father, but she forgave him. She will tell you that he didn't know better and that he did the best he could with what he knew. Maybe she's right. I know that I forgive him too. I did long before he died and for me it was cathartic. I felt lighter, as though I had let go of a huge burden, so maybe Mom was right! Is it time for me to forgive the people who have hurt me so badly?

In the book *Five Love Languages*, author Gary Chapman says, *"I have the option of justice or forgiveness, justice implies judging. With forgiveness we hope they'll do better next time."* Those are powerful words. For me, I choose to forgive the people I thought had hurt me during that dark period of my life. I choose not to grow bitter. I have apologized and now it's up to them if they choose to carry the bitterness or not. Oprah Winfrey says, *"Forgiving is letting go so the past does not hold you hostage."* I couldn't agree more.

I know there are more people Mom has forgiven: her mother for never revealing who her birth father was, her stepfather for the abuse. I could go on, but I believe the lesson here is to forgive. Just let it go. It doesn't mean that everything will be all hunky-dory just because you've forgiven someone, but you will feel better, you'll have peace of mind, and you won't walk on this beautiful earth filled with damaging anger. And that ***is*** most important.

It also doesn't mean that by forgiving, you condone what they did or that you'll reconcile with that person. No, it means you will lighten your heart and let it go. Forgiveness is a conscious, deliberate decision to release feelings of resentment toward a person who has harmed you, regardless of whether they deserve your forgiveness. You are doing this for yourself.

If you take anything away from this book, please make it about forgiveness. We need more of that in this world to lighten our hearts, our souls and forgive those who have hurt us. Whom do you need to forgive? What's stopping you? Just tell yourself, I forgive so-and-so because they did such and such, and now I will move on with my life and not think or stew on this matter any longer. You'll be glad you did – I am. Your friends will be glad too as they won't have to listen to you blather on about so-and-so any longer. It gets boring after a while hearing the same repeated gripes. Thanks, Mom, I love you. You were right.

We mustn't forget that acceptance is a very important part of forgiveness. Accepting something is not saying that it is great or that you approve of it. Acceptance is turning our suffering into pain you can endure. Your path to acceptance gets you on the road to forgiveness. Some days we ride this road, over and over again until we get it right. Once you've accepted your circumstances, then you can forgive...then you can finally heal!

To celebrate forgiveness, why not bake up a batch of Mom's Lemon Cupcakes for someone you've forgiven!

Chapter Twenty-Six

HEALING

Dear Diary,

Mom's illness and all the drama within the family are getting to me. I am crying nonstop, I am extremely nervous, I am overwhelmed and I can't sleep at night. There is a power struggle going on, some wanting this for Mom, some not. Some not wanting to get involved and others are getting implicated in imaginary offences. There are people talking to some and some not talking to others. It is a nightmare of epic proportions. Our family is falling apart right before my eyes and Mom's. Family is all she has left; and some people cannot check their egos at the door. It is shameful behavior indeed, I feel so powerless. Everyone passes Mom off as too sick to notice but I promise you, she knows all what is happening. The emotional trauma is building not just for me but many of the family, will we ever recover?

Emotional and psychological trauma can be defined as the result of extremely stressful events that destroy your sense of security, making you feel powerless in this sometimes scary world. Traumatic experiences often involve a threat to life or safety, but any situation that leaves you feeling overwhelmed and isolated can result in trauma, even if it doesn't involve physical harm. The more frightened and helpless you feel, the more likely you are traumatized.

Childhood trauma if left unchecked will carry on into adulthood and wreak havoc, setting the stage for future issues.

We all react to trauma in different ways and suffer a variety of physical and emotional symptoms. There is never a right or wrong way to think or feel, so don't judge your own reactions or those of other people. Your responses are natural reflexes to unusual events. If you've experienced the following symptoms, emotional or physical, you too likely have experienced emotional trauma: shock, denial, or disbelief are likely the first signs; even confusion and/or difficulty concentrating afterward can be exhibited. Other common symptoms would be anger, irritability, mood swings, anxiety, and fear. Are you feeling any of these symptoms? Are you feeling guilt, shame, or self-blame for things you had little or no control over? Are you feeling sad, hopeless, or numb? If you've answered yes to more than one of these, you too are likely suffering emotional trauma.

Would it surprise you to know that there are physical indicators as well to emotional trauma? For example, do you suffer insomnia or nightmares? I suffered them and still do occasionally from fatigue relating to trauma. Do you startle easily? That could be a sign of emotional trauma as well.

I have a very dear friend of mine that experiences edginess and moodiness as a result of childhood neglect and pain from bullying. Additional physical symptoms such as racing heartbeats, aches and pains, and even muscle tension affect certain people.

If you are using drugs or alcohol to deal with any of these symptoms, then please make a call and get some help. There are so many better ways to deal with your emotional trauma. Firstly, you need to allow yourself to feel what you feel when you experience it. Acknowledge your feelings about the trauma as they arise and accept them.

Healing from trauma takes time. Be patient with the pace of recovery and remember that everyone's response to trauma is different. Don't judge your loved one's reaction against your own response or anyone else's.

You may find it helps to exercise; I sure do. I like going to the gym three days a week and I prefer taking different classes. I do a Drum Zumba, muscle pump, and aerobic workouts. The classes help me engage with others. ***Exercise that is rhythmic*** and engages all your limbs, such as Zumba, running, swimming, basketball, or even dancing, works best at not only releasing endorphins but building strength and keeping you healthy.

The other exercise I enjoy very much is walking with my sweetie. We call it marriage counseling. We discuss issues while out on our evening strolls and because we're out in public, we are forced to keep it civil. Most days we walk home together but we have occasionally taken different paths back before we get too heated in our talks. Ultimately, we always sit and figure out a plan that works for both of us.

You may also want to try meditating or yoga. If you are feeling disoriented, confused, or upset, practicing deliberate breathing is a quick way to calm yourself. Simply take sixty slow and deep breaths, focusing your attention on each "out" breath. Does a specific sight, smell, or taste quickly make you feel relaxed? The smell of lavender calms me but maybe for you, it might be mint or another scent. Or maybe petting an animal or listening to music works to quickly soothe you? Everyone responds to sensory input a little differently, so experiment with different ways to find what works best for you. Personally, music is my calming method along with deep breathing, but you do what works best for you.

Both meditation and yoga are mindfulness elements you can add into your routine to deal with your emotional pain. Instead of focusing on your trauma, think about your body and how it feels in that moment. Notice how your feet feel hitting the ground, the rhythm of your breathing, the wind on your face, etc. These activities are especially helpful right before bed.

Often people like to isolate themselves from the trauma. Just engaging with people face to face will help you heal. Find comfort by simply keeping in touch with your loved ones.

You may want to participate in social activities, whether it's a weekly volleyball game, a bible study group, book club, or any other organization that may grab your attention. These are all ways to meet people and stay active in your "community." If you have no friends or live far from family, joining a group of any kind is a great way to meet people. If you've been avoiding a good friend, someone who once was important to you, take the time to reconnect. Make the effort and reach out to them.

Another fantastic way to reach out to others is by volunteering. There are so many associations that need help. Pick a group that has meaning to you. Perhaps you have strengths that you can put to use. I volunteered with "Soup Sisters" for a few years and it was so rewarding. I love making soup and I was helping the women's shelter by providing the comfort food of choice. I can tell you that I did a whole lot of healing in those times. What non-profit group can you help out while healing?

Accept the help of your loved ones. It takes a community to heal oneself and you need to allow them into your life, into your pain, into your trauma. Let them help you seek out the best professional trauma therapist for you. Meet up with the specialists and see which one is most suitable for you.

To maintain an emotional balance, you'll want to get plenty of rest. Lack of sleep can exacerbate your trauma symptoms. Try to get to bed at the same time every day and aim for seven to nine hours of sleep. It's also best to do without sleep aids or pills. Medication will work for the short term, but they are habit-forming after just ten days. When I'm having a hard time resting, I have a sleepy tea about an hour before bedtime and I sleep peacefully! I also put lavender essential oil on my pillowcase and this helps me sleep better. There are so many natural options out there for you. Do what works for you.

Eating a well-balanced diet will help you keep your energy up and minimize mood swings. Avoid sugary and fried foods and eat plenty of omega-3 fats – such as salmon, walnuts, and flaxseeds – to give your mood a boost. I like to buy different unsalted nuts (pecans, walnuts, almonds, pistachios, etc.), mix them all together in a container, and then I scoop myself a ¼ cup midafternoon snack. It gives me the little healthy boost I need to get through the rest of the day.

The most important thing you can do for yourself is to find the strength to deal with your emotional trauma once and forever. I know it feels like you don't have the energy, but believe me, you do! Even though they will all benefit, don't do it for your kids, not your husband, not your friends. Do it for yourself and do it now. You will find your life will change, you will feel healthier, and life will get so much better. I don't promise it to be an easy journey but anything worthwhile is worth doing. In order for you to heal, you have to be willing to heal. Do you really want that?

Processing trauma can be frightening, painful, and potentially re-traumatizing, so this healing work is best embarked on with the help of an experienced trauma specialist. Finding the right one may take some time. It's very important that the therapist you choose has experience treating trauma. But the quality of the relationship with your therapist is equally important. Choose a trauma specialist you feel comfortable with. If you don't feel safe, respected, or understood, find a different therapist.

There's no shame in asking for help if you're feeling overwhelmed, having trouble functioning at home or work, suffering from severe fear, anxiety, or depression. If you are experiencing terrifying memories, nightmares, or flashbacks, then perhaps it's time for you to seek a therapist, a spiritual leader or pastor, a school counselor, a doctor, or a support group. It doesn't matter who you speak to but please ***speak out*** for yourself.

I can personally attest that the heart can heal. Love yourself enough to believe that you deserve the best. You deserve peace from your pain and it can be done. Have faith; take the right steps and you too will experience gratitude, love, strength, and renewed joie-de-vivre!

Chapter Twenty-Seven

END OF AN ERA

Dear Diary,

I'm too exhausted to write Diary. I'm tired of the "he said, she said." She's this, he's that, or I did what? What nonsense! My mother is dying, and we're all worried about being right! Ugh I'm sooooo tired, I can't take much more of this. And I'm not the one lying in a bed watching it all happen. The woman spent 60 years building this family and it's all crumbling down. Give her some peace. Good night Diary, tomorrow I'll try harder to forgive. I promise.

On August 25, 2016, my sister called to tell me that Mom would be moved to Hospice. They would transfer her via ambulance to the new Hospice in Leamington. It would be a thirty-minute long bumpy ride for Mom who was in a lot of pain. They promised to dose her well before leaving.

Upon her arrival, she could not believe her room. It was beautiful, spacious, and very bright because of all the windows. They placed her in a special Lazy-boy type chair. She was enthralled with how it went up and down and she played with the remote non-stop while the nurse filled out all the forms. My sister was there with her and she thought it was funny. She hadn't seen Mom have so much fun in a long time.

Once Mom was at Hospice, I went to visit her a couple of days later; this gave my local siblings time to be with her. The drive to Leamington was just over two hours long. I put Adele in my CD player and she helped me cry. I cried for my mother's pain, I cried for myself losing my mother, for the breakdown of our families' crumbling relationship. I knew it was a just matter of time for Mom. I cried and cried, with the hopes that by the time I got there, I wouldn't cry in front of Mom. That just made Mom so sad when people cried in front of her, so I did all my crying in the car. Adele was a huge help in that way.

Once Mom got to Hospice, she was never alone. We had a little agenda book that we signed to say when we'd visit Mom. When you have seven siblings and everyone wants to be with her, it's best to schedule visits as we did. Sometimes I'd make sure I was there when my two sisters were there as they were the two siblings who supported me the most, and I did the same for them. My big brother was also supportive of me, in a quiet way and I appreciated that too. He always had a warm hug for me and still does. Mom knew there was tension in the family, and it was bothering her. She was too sick to fix anything, but she wouldn't let go until we did.

We took turns sleeping overnight in Mom's room, and it was on those nights that I'd see how Mom really was doing...and it wasn't good. My heart was broken. The woman I admired most in this world was dying a slow painful death and there was nothing I could do for her. I tried to tell her stories and kept her awake but she slept non-stop for days at a time.

On one visit, my sisters and I went into Mom's room and she was awake. We were chatting and actually got Mom to smile. We made her laugh and that was the best day for me. We have it on video as my sister was wise enough to catch that silly moment but to this day, I watch that video and smile or sometimes I cry. It's a precious memory for sure.

Mom held on for quite some time. She sensed the tension in the family and was hanging on hoping we'd all reconcile. It was her dying wish.

One day on my tear-filled ride to Leamington, I was driving through Blenheim, a small town that the highway went right through and where the speed limit would go up and down. I was caught speeding by the Chatham/Kent Police. The officer pulled me over and was not one bit friendly when I told him I was on my way to the Hospice and that I wasn't familiar with the roads in this area. He was quite short with me and proceeded to give me a $200 speeding ticket. I was so upset. It just gave me one more reason to cry with Adele and boy, did I ever. I poured my heart out to her.

I drove safely to Hospice and when I got there, I sat in the parking lot crying for I don't know how long. After collecting myself, I wiped my eyes and went into the Hospice. I couldn't believe my eyes. My long-time friend was the greeter for the day. She was a volunteer. I hugged her and cried out that she looked great, because she did, but that I looked like hell! She laughed and said that some things don't change. I hadn't seen my girlfriend in several years for no reason other than we live in different towns far from each other. Life gets busy.

I can tell you that this day was my best one at Hospice because I got to see my girlfriend again and we've since reunited in a more consistent way.

Mom lasted eight weeks at the Hospice, where they took amazing care of her. Her nurses worked tirelessly to make sure she was comfortable, always. They bathed her with such care and treated her with great dignity, kindness, and respect. I had one nurse tell me she loved Mom and I believed her. It didn't take much to love Mom because her main character in life was kindness.

Just days before Mom passed, all eight of us were gathered at the Hospice and it was Thanksgiving. They fed all of us a beautiful Thanksgiving dinner with the works: turkey, potatoes, gravy, stuffing, cranberries, pies, and they even made "pettes de soeurs," all of it. This was amazing and for a few minutes, we shared a meal and acted like a real family again. I was starting to believe we could fix this.

On this day, my sister and I talked with the older siblings. We both apologized for our part in the family drama. It was cathartic to do it and I believed we were on the right path. I felt we were going to be okay.

I stayed in the area to spend more time with Mom because I couldn't leave her. I slept a few nights at my friend's place as I didn't want to bother any of my siblings in the area as they too, were losing their mother. We were monitoring Mom closely for signs of dying, something new to me but not to my sister, unfortunately. After a few days of sleeping on a hospital bed and my friend's futon, I spoke with the duty doctor and nurses. I chose to go home to London and they promised they'd call if they caught any changes at all. Denis and I drove home and I got to have a good night's sleep in my own bed, the first one in several nights.

The next morning while grocery shopping to restock our empty cupboards, I got the call we all feared: Mom was in grave condition. We said we'd get there ASAP. This call came from a worker at the hospice, but sadly not one of my siblings.

Denis and I drove to Leamington in relative silence. Of course, I put Adele's music on, and we just listened to it. We barely spoke a word. It was a long two-hour ride and felt as if we'd never get there. At just after noon, I suddenly felt cold and out of breath. My mother had just passed and my soul knew it but I wasn't ready to accept it yet. When we got there, my sister greeted us at the back door and said to go straight into Mom's room. She told me that Mom had passed, and said, "She's still in here. Hurry, she's waiting for you."

We went in, I sobbed my little heart out. and gave my last hug to Mom. My other sister came in and the three of us hugged and had our moment. My brother came in as well, and with Denis that made five of us crying and stammering, unbelieving that at last Mom was at peace. She was no longer in pain. Nobody was ruling her or abusing her as she had suffered a lot in her life. I know she went directly to Heaven and was met by her loved ones.

After everyone had a chance to say their goodbyes to Mom, the hospice staff prepped Mom for her next journey. We created a long line on both sides of the hallway and we had an honor guard all the way out to the waiting hearse. We said a prayer, had a short ceremony, and just like that...my mother was gone.

We were told we'd get an e-mail with the service information. I was to get my eulogy ready and with that, we all hugged goodbye and went each on our way.

Days later, we arrived at the funeral home and my sister had a beautiful display of photos and flowers. There were other flowers and gifts coming in as well. We had one day of visitations, where all of Mom's friends and family came to show their respects. It was incredible how many people showed up. We had at least 500 people in attendance; those who had worked for her at the Stoney Point Tavern, people who worked with her at other jobs, friends, and neighbors. It was clear to me that Mom was loved by so many; she would've loved it because she always loved a good funeral.

I had been working on Mom's eulogy for months since I'd known long ago that I was the one to deliver it. I tweaked it after she passed and then I was ready. I prayed to God and asked him to give me the strength to not let me cry up there like a baby. I promised myself I could cry after the eulogy. I did just that and to this day am proud of the eulogy and how I delivered it.

Mom was cremated and her ashes buried with Fred. In her last days when she was able to speak still, she had asked my sister if we could bury her with Dad. My oh my, she really ***had*** forgiven him. But we knew that would never fly as Dad's wife was buried with him. She had died young of breast cancer, not long after Dad. It would've been complicated. But not to worry, some of her ashes may have slipped on Dad's grave. I think she would've said, "Well played!"

Chapter Twenty-Eight

THE EULOGY

Dear Diary,

I did it! This morning, I had prayed to God not to let me cry during my reading of the eulogy, and I made it through. I made people cry, laugh and smile. When I spoke of forgiveness and looked around at my siblings, it was not because I think they needed to forgive others but maybe they needed to forgive themselves. Maybe they needed to forgive themselves for being weak during the worst time of their life! Just let it go. Some will, some won't. All I know, it was what Mom wanted. What I never expected, was applause. The entire church clapped. It was beautiful to have a congregation applaud Mom and they did. Even the priest shared a line or two from my eulogy. I think Mom would have been proud. I miss you Mom.

"Pour nos amis et familles francophones, nous vous remercions d'être venus aujourd'hui, aussi pour vos cartes, vos dons de nourriture, vos appels, les fleurs et surtout votre soutien durant ce temps difficile.

Friends, family, and Father Dwayne. Thank you all for coming today to celebrate the life of a wonderful, exceptional woman, my Mother, Beverly Mercedes Talbot, also known as Bev Quenneville.

Mom was many things to many people. She was a daughter, a sister, a wife, first to Philippe then at a difficult time in life, she met her loyal friend Fred and they had twenty happy years together. She was a loving aunt to many, a fun friend to several, a caring boss to hundreds over the years at Stoney Point Tavern, a loving Meme or grandmother to many, a great-grandmother to even more, but most importantly to us eight siblings, she was our mother.

Mom was a loving, caring and most of all, a giving mother. She had a way to make you feel like you were her favorite. In fact, I bet all seven of my siblings would tell you that they were her favorite and truthfully they'd be right.

I asked Mom one day to tell me the truth, who was her favorite kid? She replied that at the moment I was, but she qualified that with, "But tomorrow if your sister shows up with a happy meal, she'll be my favorite, then the next day if your brother shows up to cut my lawn, he will be." You can see how this game goes, can't you? She adored all her kids and was very grateful for everything they did for her. I'm sure many of her friends would attest to that today as they were likely privy to her bragging about us, non-stop.

Mom was a Meme to many; she adored her grandkids and each of them could tell you a favorite story. You will have to ask each of them their favorite, as I can share only one today. There are many stories and I encourage you all to share them today to anybody who'll listen.

In the summer of 1993, we took Mom on a camping trip with us. She slept in our camper and on the first morning there, she took our youngest daughter, who was six at the time, to the washroom for their morning routine. They got their toothbrushes out and put their toothpaste on them, and then...we heard the laughing from our campsite! Denis and I were sitting at the site, a good distance away, and at first we thought she was crying. I ran into the washroom to see the little one and Mom laughing their fool heads off. Mom had forgotten her teeth in the camper! She was gathering a crowd and told the story over and over, breaking into laughter a few times before delivering the punch line. That weekend, Mom was known as the funny toothless Meme by everyone in the campground!

Because I lived out of town for the last 20 years, Mom and I had a standing Sunday morning phone call. In these conversations, I learned a lot about Mom's life and there was always a lesson if I listened carefully. Mom didn't have a formal post-secondary education, but she was far smarter than most people knew. It didn't take me long to figure that out.

In one of these conversations, I asked Mom, "In all your years of cooking for people, what did you like cooking the best?" Her reply was that it depended on who was showing up. She had a sense of humor too! Her one dish that shall go down in history was her chicken and glissants, or sliders. People have tried to replicate it, but I'm not convinced anyone has succeeded. Time will tell. Over the years she turned that into chicken and bow ties because it was much simpler and faster! Mom could get an unexpected meal on the table in no time at all. This is when the bow ties came in! Mom's key ingredient in everything she cooked was love. She was a fantastic cook and I am happy to tell you that she passed on many of her recipes.

On another occasion, I asked her what favorite trip she'd taken, to which she replied that it was her trip out west with my sister and her family. She said she was awed by the beauty of our country, Canada. The lesson is perhaps we should see more of our own country before we traipse all over the world. She was so grateful for the time she spent with them.

In one of our later conversations, I asked her if there was anything she wished she had done more of. She didn't hesitate to say, "Play more with my kids when they were little. I was so worried about a clean house, making the perfect dinner, being a good wife, working so much, I didn't play enough with them." There's a lesson in there for all you young moms. Meme's orders...put the mops and vacuums away!

Our phone calls came to end this past spring and we'd have our conversations face-to-face from then on. I had so many questions and knew my time was limited. I wanted to know everything about her, all her ideas, her recipes, and all her advice. She was so wise. In one of these talks, I asked her what she was most proud of in her life.

It came as no surprise to me when she answered quickly – her family. She was so proud of her eight children, how we had all found love, had wonderful children, how we are all contributing members of our society, how we were all good kids, as she put it. Family was her number one priority in life, and she felt good about the job she'd done, and she could leave us all, knowing we're all going to go on living well and passing on her traditions, morals, ethics, and her stories.

Mom was an awesome storyteller; she had a great sense of humor and had great timing. I asked her in one of our talks, which story was her favorite story to tell? She had to think as she had many, but she decided on the church and mouse story!

If you had not heard it, I will give you the Reader's Digest version. Picture our family at Sunday mass, all six kids (at the time) with Mom and Dad in a pew. She was pregnant with me; she had her winter coat on, which had just been taken out of winter storage. They were standing for prayer and she felt something run up her back. She threw off her coat and my father gave her a look. Yes, that look. Turns out there was a mouse in her coat and Dad, let's just say, took care of the mouse and handed Mom back her coat with the dead mouse inside it. She said, "No way, I'm not wearing that." So, in order not to make a scene, they switched coats. Dad wore Mom's coat home that day and Mom wore Dad's trench coat. I'll bet he looked totally handsome in that black lamb's wool coat!

On yet another trip to Belle River, I had another question. I asked her if she had any advice for us, her children. She said, "Forgive people, don't carry hate, resentment or anger, it's not good. Forgive one another." Then she used her magic little words: "Please tell them, do it for me!" Mom knew that anytime she'd use that line, no matter who she was talking to, or what she'd asked, we'd do it. She continued with, "It may be hard at times, but you'll be glad you did."

In one of our later chats, I asked Mom how she'd want to be remembered. She replied that she'd like people to remember her kindness and generosity. I assured her that would be exactly the case. I have been told exactly that by many people in the last several days. I told her that surely even a blind person could see how kind and generous she was.

I wanted to share with all of you a story today about Mom's kindness. I've been told many over this past week, so many. But the one that sticks in my mind is one a friend pointed out. She said, "With Bev, it didn't matter your race, religion, your size or color, she would be kind, loving, or funny with you as if you were her best friend." That was Mom in a nutshell, right there.

Approximately a year ago, Mom was diagnosed with Multiple Myeloma. She was about to face the battle of a lifetime, but this battle she wouldn't fight alone. Her eight kids were with her every step of the way wanting to do what they could, in whichever capacity they could. Mom faced many struggles in her lifetime, this one proved to be very daunting, but she fought nonetheless with grit, grace, and honor.

So, my friends and family, I want you to leave today not reminded of Mom's long haul of pain and suffering but of Mom's many attributes, her kindness, her generosity, her wisdom, and please carry those traits into your life. The world needs more "Bev'ness." Go out and spread the love, forgive, share, laugh and tell her stories. She'd be really happy that you did!

Mom, you made the world a better place just by being in it. We all know you are now pain-free and having the reunion of a lifetime with all your passed loved ones. We will sorely miss you.

Thank you, God bless."

Author's Closing Notes

I can't tell you how valuable it was for me to learn my family history through my chats with Mom. I don't simply mean the family tree, I mean the stories, the real-life drama of my elders' lives. After all, this information, these stories are what shaped who I am today. They shaped my mother's personality and they've shaped mine.

The stories I have shared with you are my interpretations of Mom's memoirs to me. I'm certain that others in the family will have a different version of the same events and hopefully, someday they'll write their own book, which would be totally acceptable with me.

My hope is that you've garnered a lesson or two from our past mistakes. Forgiveness is the lesson I gained most from Mom. If she could forgive people for the way she was treated for most of her life, then surely I can forgive those that have hurt me. I hope you can too. If you need help with that, please reach out to me.

If I've stirred memories for you, I want to suggest to you that maybe it's time to move forward and leave all that in the past. Perhaps it's time to forgive the past, make peace with it, and start fresh.

I want to acknowledge that even though we've forgiven our offenders, it is no guarantee that they will change or have changed. Not everyone on this earth is necessarily meant to be a part of our lives, even if you are related. We need to set boundaries and we determine who we let within those boundaries.

Lastly, as you can tell, food is always a part of our story. I am very much a foodie as was my mother. I'd like to give you a link to all the recipes and food I mention in the book. Follow this link to your free recipes!

www.themonkeysinmydreams.com

About The Author

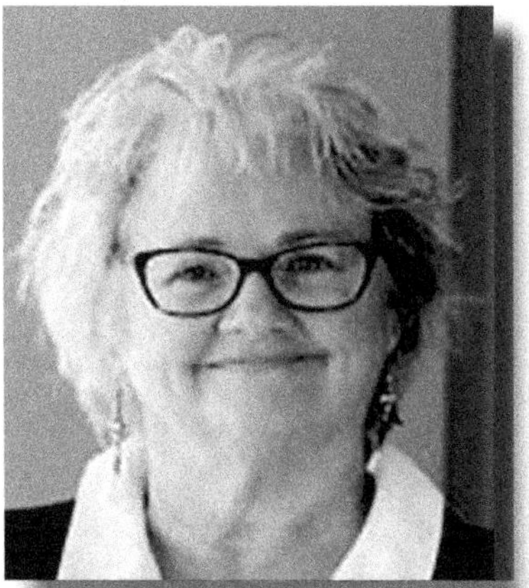

Anne-Marie Bacon grew up in a large family. She was the seventh child of eight, born to Bev and Phil. Anne-Marie is the blessed daughter of Beverley, a woman who bravely shared all of her deep, dark secrets. With those stories, Anne-Marie weaved the story of *The Monkeys in My Dreams – Healing Generational Trauma Through Love, Hope & Forgiveness.*

Anne-Marie has been happily married for thirty-nine years to Denis and together they have raised two smart and beautiful daughters. Those lovely girls have had two children each, so a total of four grandchildren keep Anne-Marie and Denis young and happy! Spending time with their grandchildren has been both educational and entertaining.

When not writing, Anne-Marie and Denis love to travel where they immerse themselves in the local culture, food, and surroundings. They are partial to the warm sunshine of Mexico to escape the cold, brutal winter of Southern Ontario, Canada but have been known to frolic in Europe as well.

Anne-Marie has been on the path to healing and forgiveness for some time now. Writing this book gave her much fodder, hearing all of her mother's stories and her ease to forgive. She recently completed the course for a Certified Life Coach which gave her an entirely new perspective in healing. Her journey continues daily.

Have a question for Anne-Marie? Please contact her at:
monkeysinmydreams@outlook.com

CPSIA information can be obtained
at www.ICGtesting.com
Printed in the USA
BVHW040102020521
606281BV00001B/1

9 781988 867359